COPING WITH STROKE

Helen Broida

College-Hill Press, 4580-E Alvarado Canyon Road, San Diego, California 92120

Library of Congress Cataloging in Publication Data
Broida, Helen
    Communication breakdown of brain injured adults.
    (coping with stroke)
    Bibliography: p.
    Includes index.
    1. Aphasics—Rehabilitation. 2. Speech, Disorders of. 3. Brain Damage—Complications and sequelae. 4. Communicative disorders. I. Title. [DNLM: 1. Aphasia—Popular works. 2. Brain injuries, Acute—Popular works. 3. Communication—Popular works. WL354 B866c]
    RC425.B75   616.8'552   79-220
    ISBN 0-933014-50-3

Printed in the United States of America

TO
Vicki, Ronna, and Shaw

CONTENTS

Preface

When I began to treat adult aphasic patients, I longed for a book to give me guidelines for answering questions posed by their concerned family members. No such book was available. I had consumed the required textbooks for speech pathology graduate students that discussed language function in relation to brain mechanisms, neurological disorders, phonetics, linguistics, and all the rest, but these learned texts were of small value when face to face with the families of aphasic-apraxic-dysarthric patients who looked to me for guidance. My training as a marriage and family counselor did not necessarily prepare me for guiding a family in a particular kind of crisis, shocked by the catastrophic intrusion of brain injury to a husband or wife, parent, son, or daughter, yet needing to make sometimes immediate far-reaching decisions concerning some very pressing practical problems. Often I was the only professionally trained person remaining in regular, frequent contact with them, because language therapy continues long after other therapies have reached their full treatment potential and long after a physician is required to follow a patient closely. There were and are a variety of pamphlets available, each of special value, but all limited in their scope, so that few families can find enough of their own needs met in reading them; therefore, families naturally often turn to the speech pathologist for guidance.

In my contacts with nurses, occupational and physical therapists, vocational rehabilitation counselors, social workers, and even some physicians, I found that there were serious misconceptions of what some of our shared aphasic patients could really understand and of how functional was their total language capability. I wished for a book to which I could refer them that would delineate communication dysfunctioning in a non-academic fashion, so that they had some means of screening the reliabiity, for example, of a patient's "yes" or "no" when asked a vital question concerning his past health history. No such book was available.

As supervisor of clinical training of graduate students in speech pathology, I have long wished for a book to supplement academic readings, a book to provide discussion and some solutions to frequent, practical, daily concerns in the lives of their brain injured, communication disordered patients. I could not find such a book.

These are the gaps I have tried to fill with this book. However, because it has been written to make similar information available to several groups of people whose needs for it differ somewhat, it has been necessary in the writing to find common denominators so that some presentations may appear too sketchy for one group, too technical for another, and regretably perhaps, redundant.

In the preparation of this manuscript, I am indeed grateful for the suggestions of Jean Weissman Richlin, Milton Richlin, David Price, Thomas Murry, Nancy Douglas, Lynn Mohns, Frieda Gendloff, Judy Bugbee, and Sally Kreger, each of whom brought expertise from different backgrounds or disciplines and helped to pull me back when I went astray. Perhaps I resisted their pull now and then through these pages when I should have submitted, but their assistance throughout has been of strong value to me.

Helen Broida, Ph.D.
Speech Pathologist

Foreword

When first approached with the request to prepare an introduction to this volume, I must confess to some misgivings. It was only after having had an opportunity to read the manuscript that I began to appreciate how consistent the views of the author are with my own. After discovering this, I attacked the problem with considerable enthusiasm. Dr. Broida reflects in a very practical and specific way the need to introduce into the rehabilitation program of any adult with a communication disorder resulting from brain injury, those elements which are normally in that person's environment. In consideration of this, the family becomes particularly important. A great deal is sacrificed when the family is not brought into the picture and made to appreciate exactly what is going on. Furthermore, there are not enough therapists nor is there enough money to solve these problems without taking advantage of all the ingredients and using them to the fullest extent possible.

While the immediate concern of the language therapist in dealing with the adult suffering from a communication disorder is the reacquisition of language, the recovery of that individual rests with the total reintegration of physical structure, medical condition, personality, and intellect. Language should not be considered as a separate and independent therapeutic need since it is only within an integrated framework that one can view language therapy.

Clearly, many individuals are not prepared either physically or mentally for more than supportive therapy during the initial phase following brain injury. Furthermore, one must remember that it is during this period that one should anticipate that spontaneous recovery of function may take place. It is not infrequent to find during the early post-acute stage that a totally unrealistic sense of well-being pervades the attitude of the patient. The functional disability, which is so obvious to the examiner, has little or no importance for the person affected. One cannot induce changes from outside during this period and such change as may occur results from the continuing alteration of the patient's neurologic status. It is during this period that more cortical neurons may become available for integrative function. In addition, it is common to observe during the early recovery phase extreme emotional lability which may produce in the patient a catastrophic response to whatever inquiry is made or whatever task the person is requested to fulfill. The three most important factors which must be considered in language therapy are: 1) stimulation, 2) facilitation, and 3) motivation. In more simple terms these consist of what the therapist does, what the cerebral cortex in an injured state is capable of doing, and what level of acceptance the patient has achieved in his or her progress toward recovery. The immediate goal of the therapist must always be to work toward change, to stimulate the injured person only slightly above his or her ability of the moment while not getting so far out in front that the individual loses sight of realistic goals. It is clear from this volume that therapy in the adult with a communication disorder requires the utmost in ingenuity. It can never be routine, predetermined, or automated because language deficits are complex. Therapy for them is equally complex, and there is always a need for individualization with a program designed to suit the needs and capabilities of each brain injured person. No matter how the program is structured it is full of frustration for the patient, for the therapist, and above all, for the family.

Unlike many authors on the subject of language therapy who have presented "carefully designed formulas" for the management of brain injured individuals, Dr. Broida in her text brings into better focus the emotional and intellectual considerations in the rehabilitation of the brain injured adult with communication disorder. She points out that treatment requires cooperation and active participation on the part of the affected individual who must, above all, adjust, understand, and accept treatment. She recognizes that the patient's emotional and intellectual stata can readily influence the final outcome of the rehabilitation effort. It becomes very clear that such factors as premorbid emotional, intellectual, educational, occupational, and social stata contribute in large measure to the post-injury patterns and more particularly, the rehabilitation potential. When the brain injured individual first becomes aware of the physical and communicative limitations which have been brought about by the injury, the immediate reaction is always partly determined by the premorbid psychological make-up. One must deal with several frequently encountered emotional patterns such as acute depression, marked emotional lability, withdrawal, states of over-anxiety, euphoria, and conspicuous alterations in mood. Communicative impairment will often intensify these behavioral abnormalities which may vary greatly from hour to hour and day to day, most often in the acute stage and remain until the patient's condition has become stabilized.

Communicative disorder may produce not only abrupt but devastating change in the patient's lifestyle and some of the aforementioned emotional and adaptive responses are the overt manifestations of this change. One must face the fact, however, that the brain damage itself may produce psychopathologic changes and it clearly becomes very important to determine which behaviors are attributable to the brain damage and which are not. Furthermore, some emotional and adaptive behaviors, such as anxiety when kept under reasonable control, may play a vital role in establishing and maintaining motivation. Therefore, as is pointed out by the author, one must determine which reaction patterns may be looked upon as assets and which must be minimized in order to avoid interference with the management program.

The patient's intellectual capability must be assessed in a manner which will assist in determining whether or not there will be benefit from practice and transference of what has been achieved in one task to other slightly more complex ones. The therapist must be constantly testing experimentally the manner and the rate in which behavior changes. This type of approach does not take into consideration intelligence in the conventional sense, but it may tell us a great deal more about what the individual can do with the available intellectual potential than those tests which, up to now, have been most frequently employed. Dr. Broida is very careful to point out that one should not be hasty in making judgments about intellectual impairment until the closest possible contact has been made with the impaired individual. If it can be determined that an individual has the intellectual capacity and psychological make-up required to provide a base upon which to build reintegration to a satisfactory social status, it should then be possible to establish the level of available psycholinguistic ability.

Dr. Broida, as a result of the length and breadth of her experience, has come to recognize that the therapeutic challenge of the adult with communication difficulty lies not only in the ability of the language therapist, but with a team effort always designed to include the patient's family. She points out that the goals of therapy should not be expressed only in terms of verbal elements, which can be received, integrated and expressed, but rather in terms of the patient regaining the ability to communicate in specific life situations which may be encountered in the future. For example, in the section devoted to sexual behavior in the brain injured adult, she addresses a very important subject which physicians need to understand and also to appreciate how important it is for them to counsel both the spouse and the patient before the latter is dismissed from direct care. Unfortunately, far too many people think that sex is a taboo after brain injury and are fearful of shocking their physicians by even bringing the matter to their attention. This book provides for the layman the only available information on this subject of which I am aware.

This book will be a valuable asset to physicians, nurses, occupational and physical therapists, vocational rehabilitation counselors, social workers, graduate students of speech pathology, and practicing speech therapists. The manner in which it is presented provides a very efficient design for rapid location of responses to many perplexing questions.

William S. Fields, M.D.
Houston, Texas

Chapter I

Introduction

Aphasia is the name given to a language disturbance caused by brain damage. Aphasia, one of the most frightening conditions that can befall a human being. And it is almost as staggering a blow to the family as it is to the person suffering the disorder.

We learn to communicate at a very early age. We grow up taking for granted that we will always be able to understand what is said in our native tongue (if it concerns subjects within our range of knowledge), that we will always be able to tell others what we wish to say to them and to read and write adequately enough for our needs. Some among us have developed communication skills to a higher level of competence than others, but most of us can use language to exchange information with others satisfactorily. Unless we become aphasic.

The person stricken with aphasia may suddenly be unable to find words that he wants to say. Without warning, everyone around him, simultaneously, may appear to be speaking in a foreign language because he may be unable to understand a word others are saying. Newspapers and books may appear to be covered with undecipherable squiggles. Attempts to write may produce only meaningless scrawls, because spelling, letters, grammar and the words themselves may be lost, temporarily or permanently, depending upon the extent of the damage. To the individual affected, the loss of communication is indeed a terrifying and isolating state, and the trauma to the family is devastating.

At the onset the physician is the key person to whom the family turns. Survival is the central issue of this early period and that, of course, is a medical concern. When it becomes evident that the patient is going to survive, then the growing anxiety of the family centers on residual impairments. Will they clear up? Will they require treatment? What kinds? What will the cost be? What can family and friends do to help? What should they *not* do?

These and many more questions emerge but often the family does not know whom to ask or where to find the answers. Physicians are busy and many families are timid about approaching a medical doctor with non-medical questions. Indeed, many physicians do not have answers to specific questions about treatment of aphasia or other communication problems, since this is the province of the speech pathologist who is trained in testing and therapy for speech and language problems following brain damage.

One purpose for this book is to answer many of the questions families want answered—to clarify for the family what is known today about aphasia and other communication disorders, what treatment should be pursued and when, by whom and for how long, what goals can be considered realistic, and how to cope with the multitude of other difficulties created by the impairment of a family member. Many anxieties can be alleviated by knowing what and what not to do, and even by becoming fully aware that for most patients the former skills and conditions of living will not completely return. We human beings are far better able to handle sadness than we are anxiety, and although knowing the truth may bring with it much sadness, release from the anxiety of not knowing often results in better ability to cope.

This book can also be helpful to paramedicals who see patients with communication disorders but do not quite know how to communicate with some of them, and in what ways they might enhance the time spent with these patients by including techniques that can help the language difficulties. I am often asked by nurses, physical and occupational therapists, social workers and others if there are specific things they might do, or should not do, while working with such patients. My reply is always an enthusiastic affirmative. Everyone who is in a position to communicate with the patient can contribute to progress by knowing what can help and what should be avoided.

Students of speech pathology who want to treat brain damaged adults should find this book to be informative, augmenting information gleaned from textbooks on speech and language disorders. Textbooks rarely, if ever, deal with the living problems of stricken adults and their families. The speech pathologist often becomes the only professional in long-term, frequent contact with the patient, and therefore is the one the family is most likely to approach for advice and direction with problems that are decidedly not textbook problems.

Since some physicians see aphasic patients only in the acute stages of the disorder, many do not know that even years after onset significant numbers of aphasics are capable of improving their communicative ability if they receive proper language therapy. This book provides physicians with a viewpoint of diagnosis, treatment, and prognosis that can be helpful.

Due to the enormous complexity of speech and language there are many types of speech and language disorders. Although this book will attempt to deal with questions most frequently asked, none are necessarily applicable to all patients. Therefore, the book is divided into chapters, each dealing with a specific aspect of various difficulties. Chapters are listed in the Contents along with the questions pertaining to that particular aspect of the disorder and the page where the response is provided. The reader, therefore, should be able to locate those questions and answers with which he is concerned, and if he chooses, ignore discussions that do not fit his circumstances.

Throughout the book, except in sections specifically directed toward women, the patient is referred to as "he." The need to use a pronoun is obviously a matter of simplifying the presentation. The pronoun selected chould just as easily have been "she." There is no sexism involved in the final choice.

Chapter II

General Information About Stroke and Other Causes of Brain Damage

What is a Stroke?
What is the Importance of Brain Cells?
How Common Are Strokes in the United States?
How Many Deaths in This Country Are Due to Strokes?
Do Many Stroke Victims Recover with No Permanent Damage?
Are There Warnings Before a Stroke Occurs?
In What Ways Does Communication Break Down After a Stroke?
Why is Paralysis Limited to One Side or the Other After a Stroke?
Do Other Causes of Brain Damage Produce the Same Results as Stroke?
Is Memory Affected by Brain Damage?
Why do Some Brain Injured People Laugh or Cry at Strange, Inappropriate Times?
Has the Brain Damaged Person "Lost His Mind"?
Should Others Do Things for the Brain Injured Person That He Can Do for Himself?

What Is a Stroke?

The technical name for stroke is cerebral vascular accident or CVA. "Cerebral" refers to the brain which is where a stroke takes place. "Vascular" refers to the blood vessels. A stroke results when the blood supply feeding the brain cells is cut off from those cells by an "accident" to the blood vessels through which the blood circulates. Many people are surprised to learn this, not realizing that strokes and heart attacks can have much in common and can often be caused by the same problem depending on the location of the vascular accident. The most common cause of a CVA is a blockage of one of the arteries supplying blood to a section of the brain, a blockage due to thickening of the walls of the artery thus narrowing the channel through which the blood flows (thrombosis), or to a traveling clot (embolism) that becomes lodged in one of the arteries.

Another cause of stroke is cerebral hemorrhage or a bursting of an artery in the brain. When this occurs the brain cells fed by that artery do not receive their necessary nourishment so they cannot function. Furthermore, the blood that hemorrhages can cause damage by the force of its emission, and the cumulation of blood that floods the surrounding area interferes with the functioning of that part of the brain. Until the blood and other fluids caused by the hemorrhage are absorbed and the uninjured cells resume functioning, the actual amount of damage cannot be determined. This absorption can take several months.

What Is the Importance of Brain Cells?

Brain cells are nerve cells that control most of our muscular movements, our sensations, our speech and other language, our thinking, our memory, indeed, our entire ability to function in the world. When brain cells fail, the body parts or other activity they control cannot function. Whether the resulting disability will be temporary or permanent, mild or severe, depends upon how widespread the nerve cell damage is, which cells are damaged, and how effectively the body can repair the blood supply to those parts.

A damaged brain cell, unlike nerve cells in other parts of the body, does not seem to regenerate; at least that has long been the conclusion drawn by scientists who work with the brain. Lately some reports are emerging that may change these opinions. Damage to brain cells is what is meant when the term "brain damage" is used. There are those who say we are all brain damaged to some extent as all of us lose some brain cells along the way.

How Common Are Strokes in the United States?

There are about two and one half million people in the United States today who have had strokes; 500,000 new stroke cases are reported in this country annually. Among whites the incidence of strokes is 2 to 1 of men to women, and among blacks it is 3 to 2.

How Many Deaths in This Country are Due to Stroke?

Stroke is the third largest cause of death in the United States at this time, exceeded only by heart attack and cancer. The figure reported by the National Institute of Neurological and Communicative Disorders and Stroke is 200,000 deaths annually due to stroke. More strokes are caused by thrombosis and embolism than by hemorrhage, and many more people survive the former two than survive hemorrhage.

Do Many Stroke Victims Recover with No Permanent Damage?

Unfortunately, only about 10 percent of people who survive strokes can return to their accustomed life-styles with virtually no residual impairment. However, 40 percent suffer only mild disability with little interference in their way of life *unless they choose to let it interfere.* Another 40 percent are disabled enough to require special services such as physical therapy, occupational therapy, speech and language therapy, vocational rehabilitation, etc. The remaining 10 percent will be so severely disabled as to require permanent institutional care.

Are There Warnings Before a Stroke Occurs?

Yes, for some people. These are called transient ischemic attacks (TIAs). They may occur weeks before an actual stroke. They occur in any form a stroke can take: a sudden weakness or even paralysis of a part of the body, an inability to speak, loss of sensation of a body part, and so on. They are transient, fleeting episodes. Full function is restored within 24 hours. Tragically, many people ignore these warning signs of impending trouble. What their bodies are signalling is that an artery is briefly clogged, shutting off nourishment from a group of brain cells although not long enough to do actual damage to them. A few weeks later the same clogging may recur without reversing itself, and a stroke results.

The brief episode should not have been ignored. This is the time to see a physician. Immediately! At this time there are often, although not always, steps a physician can take that may prevent a full stroke. Stroke prevention is of utmost importance because death or permanent disability are such frequent consequences of strokes.

In What Ways Does Communication Break Down After a Stroke?

The language center of the brain of most people is in the left hemisphere. When damage occurs to the portion of the left side of the brain that controls language, a communication disorder results that is known as *aphasia*. There is a small percentage of people whose language centers are in the right hemisphere. These people may become aphasic if the right side of their brain is damaged in the language area.

Aphasia may encompass all the ways in which we communicate with each other. It includes disruption in ability to understand the speech of others, to speak with the correct words and grammar, to read, to write, and to use gestures meaningfully. Computing, arithmetic, and telling time are usually also disturbed. In some cases only one of these language skills is disrupted; more often some degree of difficulty is experienced in most or all skills when someone develops aphasia.

The aphasic's speech difficulty is generally the most obvious problem but the family is often unaware that he may understand very little of what is said, especially if he smiles and nods when they speak to him as so many aphasic patients do with what seems to be good comprehension. It may be some time before even the patient learns that he has difficulty reading and writing, because in the early stages he may have no desire or need to try these skills.

When the brain cells controlling the muscles needed to produce speech or voice are injured on either side of the brain, speech is likely to be slurred and the voice may be hoarse, nasal, or breathy. The pitch may be uncontrolled or monotone. These conditions are not part of aphasia although they may exist along with it. They are part of a speech disorder known as *dysarthria*. In dysarthria words and grammar are not lost, but the muscles needed to utter the words properly or to produce the voice have been weakened or paralyzed by damage to the brain cells controlling these muscles. The dysarthria may be so slight that the patient is understood as well as ever but sounds a bit different, or it can be so severe that he cannot be understood at all. Since the same muscles used for speech and voice quality are also used for swallowing and eating, some dysarthric patients must be fed through tubes. Dysarthrics may drool because of the muscular weakness and there may also be a sensory loss so they cannot feel the moisture accumulating.

Another communication disorder that can exist alone or with aphasia and dysarthria is called *apraxia of speech*. In apraxia the muscles are not weakened or paralyzed as in dysarthria, nor has the apraxic person forgotten the word as in aphasia. Instead he has forgotten how to place his tongue, lips, and mouth in the correct positions and to sequence these positions in the right order to produce the desired word, phrase, or sentence. The apraxic person may produce some perfectly intact automatic phrases which may or may not be appropriate, but when he tries volitionally to say something, his struggle to approach the correct pronunciation can be painful to observe. If the word is spoken, giving him a model to imitate, he will have difficulty imitating the model. The aphasic who is not also apraxic will have no difficulty imitating. The dysarthric will be consistently unable to produce certain sounds correctly, so if the model presented contains these sounds he will utter a distortion of the word. When a patient is aphasic, dysarthric, and apraxic the problems are compounded greatly and are difficult to sort out. Since each condition requires a different treatment it is desirable to sort them out if possible.

Right-handed people have a dominant left hemisphere and a non-dominant right hemisphere. When right-handed people incur damage to their non-dominant right hemisphere, there are often changes in their use of language, although they will not be aphasic. They may become very talkative and use flowery, eloquent language very different from their habitual mode of expression. They may have difficulty reading because they may have spatial-perceptual deficits that cause them to keep losing their place on a page. These same deficits may cause writing problems. These patients may be difficult to deal with because their judgment is often poor and they may attempt to do things, even dangerous things, that they are completely unable to do.

Why Is Paralysis Limited to One Side or the Other After a Stroke?

The muscles on one side of the body are controlled by the nerve cells in the opposite half or hemisphere of the brain. Because of the nature of the blood supply to the brain, a stroke generally occurs in one hemisphere or the other in any one incident (unless it is in the brain stem which creates still other kinds of problems). There may be a succeeding stroke causing damage in the other side of the brain also, but as a rule only one side is affected by a single stroke. If a stroke damages an area of the left hemisphere including the nerve cells that control the right arm and leg, these limbs will be paralyzed or weakened depending upon the extent of the damage. If they are paralyzed, this is called right *hemiplegia*. If they are weakened the condition is called right *hemiparesis*. Since the language centers are nearby in the same hemisphere, that person may very likely have aphasia also. Sometimes hemiplegia improves to become hemiparesis, especially if physical therapy has been administered. Some patients can regain sufficient use of their legs to walk with a limp but often do not regain use of a paralyzed arm.

Other muscle groups along the right side, such as the muscles of the face, mouth, and tongue, usually will be affected. There may a drooping of the right side of the face, a slurring of speech (dysarthria), and perhaps some drooling.

Since sensation may be affected by nerve cell damage, some of these problems may be due to lack of feeling in the parts involved so that signals are not sent back to the brain to inform that organ of what is going on. The patient who drools may not be aware of the moisture on his chin because he cannot feel it on that side. To the onlooker, unaware of this possibility, it appears that he does not care that he is drooling. In fact, however, many stroke patients become very distraught when they see in a mirror what has happened.

When a stroke occurs in the right hemisphere, the paralysis will be on the left side of the body and all the above described conditions may exist on that side, but in most people there will be no aphasia. There might, however, be the type of language problems discussed earlier that are found when the non-dominant hemisphere is affected.

Do Other Causes of Brain Damage Produce the Same Results as Stroke?

Any head injury can lead to brain cell damage and a damaged nerve cell no longer controls that function for which it exists. Thus aphasia can be produced by a fall from a ladder, an automobile accident, a hang-glider or motorcycle crash. Brain tumors, either benign or malignant, can interfere with brain cell functioning and may do irreversible damage. Surgery itself, anywhere in the body, provides a potential risk for brain damage by releasing a blood clot or by surgical shock. Although any of these causes can produce aphasia, dysarthria, apraxia, muscle weakness, paralysis, or loss of sensation, the pattern of the disabilities differs from the pattern following stroke. This is because the area of the brain damaged by stroke depends upon the nature of the blood supply to that area, whereas in accidents, tumors, or surgical causes the damage is random, depending upon the areas stricken. Damage from other causes is frequently more widespread than damage from stroke, often involving both hemispheres. If the brain cells controlling arms and legs are involved the person may be *quadriplegic* which means all four limbs are paralyzed. He may not only have aphasia but also the problems of spatial relationships and other difficulties that arise when the non-dominant hemisphere is damaged.

The pattern of disability with brain tumor depends upon the location and size of the tumor and what brain cells it is disturbing. Surgery may successfully remove some tumors so that there are few or no residuals, but in other cases surgery itself can do some damage. In tumor the onset of behavior changes is not sudden as in stroke or accidents, but usually develops so gradually that symptoms may go unnoted until the tumor has progressed far.

The course of improvement in accident and tumor cases differs from stroke. The latter is more apt to have a predictable rate of spontaneous improvement (see Chapter III). Other causes of brain damage do not lend themselves to prediction of improvement very comfortably.

Is Memory Affected by Brain Damage?

Many people who suffer even very mild brain damage find they have trouble remembering things that happened a short time earlier, although they clearly recall events that took place years ago. Short term or recent memory is often affected by brain damage, just as it is often found to be a problem in the normal aging process of many people.

If the family and others involved with the patient realize that memory can be faulty following the onset of brain injury and may continue to be faulty from then on, many frustrations may be avoided. When something important needs to be carried out by someone who has suffered brain damage, a check list or some other form of reminder should be provided, rather than reliance on his memory of a verbal request. It is important for the patient to become as independent as his condition will allow; however, it is also important that he does not forget critical matters, such as those pertaining to health, for example, regular medication. Care should be taken to prevent him from experiencing repeated failures due to memory impairment that could easily have been avoided by good planning. If and when he is able to assume responsibilities which he might forget, an open, honest discussion of his "tricky" memory needs to be held and solutions proposed. In some cases the only solution is that someone else always assumes that particular responsibility.

Depending upon the patient's personality, life-long habits, and the character of his brain damage, his reaction to his memory problem will vary. An actress, such as Patricial Neal (Farrel, 1969) who suffered a brain hemorrhage when she was three months pregnant, apparently was deeply disturbed by her poor memory. Obviously, unless her memory improved there was no way she would ever be able to memorize lines again should she return to her profession. Time has shown she recovered both memory and speech well enough to resume her acting career very satisfactorily. If there is damage to the non-dominant side of the brain, the patient may deny that he has a problem. Some will insist they were never told what to do; others, that they actually accomplished it. Many a family battle has been provoked by such situations. Wives or husbands have complained: "There's nothing wrong with his (her) memory! It's just stubbornness. He (she) remembers in detail everything that happened in business (or a dinner party) 20 years ago, but can't remember to do a simple thing like turn on the oven at 3 PM so we can have dinner when I come home from work. He (she) expects me to do everything!"

When these family members become aware that there is a vast difference between long-term, stored memories and recently acquired memories, and that the latter typically can become faulty with brain damage, the anger and frustration following such episodes can be so relieved that solutions are often just waiting there to be discovered. A casual phone call at 3 PM, perhaps seemingly just to touch base and say hello, and an innocent inquiry about the oven, might be just the way to handle it with some people. With others it might be better to use humor, making light of the memory failure but providing the reminder.

When brain damage is more extensive, long-term memory can also be impaired. Even familiar faces can be forgotten. It is good to keep in mind that in the early weeks after onset there are many impairments that will improve, and severe memory deficiencies may well be part of this.

Another aspect of memory that can become faulty with brain damage is the *retention span*. This refers to the number of "pieces of information" a person can retain at one time. For example, the normal adult can usually handle a message like this: "Dinner is ready. Please call the children, turn off the TV, and see that everyone washes his hands." This message contains four separate elements or pieces of information to be acted upon. To the brain damaged person who can understand each part of this message if given alone or with not more than one other part of the message, the four elements may be an overload. This means he may become confused and not retain any of the message at all, or shut out all of it after "Dinner is ready." When he then appears at the table without the children, who are still watching television, an emotional situation may be precipitated that could well have been avoided if the retention span limitations were understood. When the brain damaged person has a retention span limited to two elements, no more than two at a time should ever be given.

How is the length of the retention span determined? If there is no speech pathologist available who can test this, the best way is trial and error with the following techniques. Start with one-element messages, such as "Point your finger." When it is certain that several of these simple messages are carried out well individually, combine two of the elements into one statement on another day. Only when a series of two-element messages are easily acted upon over a period of several days should a third one be added in the same way. If, however, there is a fluctuation in ability to act upon both elements in a two-part message so that: (1) sometimes they are completed and other times one is forgotten, or (2) confusion sets in and both are lost or only one is ever carried out, or (3) an incorrect act is substituted, then a third element should not be added. Even two should be given with care.

Perhaps he will never be able to handle more than two, and dependably, never more than one. As hard as this information is to accept by family members, it will eventually produce a more peaceful home environment when this type of information is understood, accepted, and dealt with properly.

Why Do Some Brain Injured People Laugh or Cry at Strange, Inappropriate Times?

Brain damage often produces emotional *lability* which is another way of saying emotional instability. Any one of us who has been through debilitating illness or surgery has perhaps experienced the type of poor emotional controls accompanying general weakness of the body. Labile behavior following brain damage may be due to this weakness in some people; as they get stronger they develop better control over laughter and tears. However, brain damage itself can destroy or temporarily inhibit the controls we normally have over laughing and crying. Thus the strong man may weep when someone praises his effort, to the embarrassment of friends and family who do not understand that this can be a normal consequence of brain damage. He may also laugh heartily at his failures or at what should be treated as sad or serious news. Others, then, may become angered at his "callousness." There are some patients who appear to be happy all the time, in spite of a very severe disablement. This is a condition of *euphoria* caused by brain damage; it can be very disturbing to those who read it as supreme indifference to the burden his condition has placed upon them.

How to deal with "inappropriate" laughter, tears, or happiness? The first step is to try to understand the situation. The observer sees nothing that should have produced any of these reactions; therefore, the word "inappropriate" is, so to speak, in the eye of the beholder. It is tempting to read meanings into lability, and to try to console or to scold according to the interpretation one has reached. No one can really know why each person laughs or cries at such times, nor can anyone understand what the euphoric patient is comprehending of his present status. Even the patient himself may not know. Some patients feel extremely foolish when they cannot shut off their laugher or tears; they feel diminished by such behavior. Therapists have found that ignoring the laughter or tears is the best way of helping. Say nothing. Do nothing. Try to procede as if it were not taking place. If this is not possible while the emotional state is in evidence, then busying oneself with some other activity until the episode has passed is best. Unless the brain damage is very extensive and the physical weakness extremely debilitating, time should provide better controls, for some, even a return to normal emotional functioning.

As for euphoria, surely this is a better consequence than overwhelming anger and withdrawal, which some patients do exhibit. It is probable that the patient who is euphoric does not fully grasp the significance of his disability. If there is damage in the non-dominant hemisphere, it is very possible that he totally denies to himself that any change has occurred.

Has the Brain Damaged Person "Lost His Mind"?

Many families fear that the person who suffers brain damage is now mentally incompetent or psychotic because his speech and behavior are so different from what they were. This is not likely to be the case, unless damage was very extensive. When the dominant hemisphere (usually the left) is involved and aphasia develops, the disturbance in language does not mean that the patient is impaired intellectually. When he is able to understand what is said, his judgment may be as good as it ever was. He may be labile temporarily, as discussed earlier, and he may be saddened by his impairment. This is certainly a normal reaction. But the concept of "loss of mind" in our society usually means either insanity or mental retardation. Brain injury does not necessarily cause either of these.

When the non-dominant hemisphere (usually right) is involved, certain personality changes take place that may impair judgment and reliability. These changes must be recognized and taken into consideration when the patient is involved in decision making. But this does not imply that he is psychotic or retarded.

If he displays dangerous behavior or a marked loss of intellectual ability so that he is *demented*, the physician can often determine this and will include it in his diagnosis. Everyone should have a fairly good idea whether either of these conditions exists long before the patient is ready to leave the hospital, because his behavior in the hospital would have made it apparent.

Dementia means a combination of deteriorated thinking, inability to remember, lack of emotional control, totally incorrect and sometimes even dangerous use of certain objects, impaired judgment, and impaired orientation to people, place, and time. The demented person might try to eat his comb instead of combing his hair. He might turn on the gas without lighting it, and use the shower as a toilet. Some of this behavior is found in patients with *sensory or ideational apraxia* who do not recall the nature and purpose of objects. A combination of traits, not just one group, is necessary for a diagnosis of dementia. There are qualitative and quantitiative differences between dementia and other forms of brain damaged behavior. The physician or speech pathologist can help differentiate.

Even patients who display demented behavior early after onset may sometimes become better integrated and intellectually adequate again. If they are aphasic as well, speech therapy may have an integrative effect upon their intellectual functioning, helping to normalize them.

A woman in her early forties, mother of three small children, brought her husband to me for evaluation nearly three years after he had become aphasic due to Herpes Encephalitis. They had been living where no speech therapy was available until their recent move to the west coast. She was almost beside herself with anxiety and conflict. Her husband had no apparent physical disability, but he seemed to understand nothing that was said to him and his speech was almost complete jargon, interspersed with bursts of laughter. He frequently wandered away from home so that often she had to bundle up her three children and systematically hunt for him, driving slowly up and down all the nearby streets. She resisted placing him into a locked facility because, as she put it, he had been a wonderful husband and father until this tragedy struck. Now he was like a child, needing constant surveillance, but she hated the thought of putting him away from his family. Yet their oldest child seemed to show signs of resenting and even being ashamed of him. He was eneuretic and sometimes incontinent of bowels. He did strange things, she said, put things into his mouth that were not meant for eating. A few times he had started a fire in the kitchen.

My evaluation was to be the crucial element in her decision regarding placement. The test showed that he probably could function at a higher level in language, even significantly higher, but the demented type of behavior and the bilateral damage were such that it seemed unlikely that he could improve in those areas. However, his wife wanted a trial period of therapy if there was any chance of improvement, so with misgivings it was undertaken.

The results were very gratifying. Within the trial period, he began to understand much that was said to him he stopped running away, and after another month the incontinence ended completely. It was a joyful day when she knew she did not have to place him away from home. In a few more months he became so trustworthy that she was able to send him to school to pick up the children, saving her much needed time to accomplish other errands. There was a slight tendency remaining to use some materials inappropriately for a while; then he went through a period where he quickly corrected himself when he began these incorrect actions; and finally the sensory apraxia vanished completely. He was found to be severely apraxic of speech so that it took many months before he was able to imitate anything, but after two years of speech therapy, he finally learned to say some important words and short sentences, including the names of his children and his wife, with great pride. His wife said often, "Speech therapy has given my husband back to me."

The demented patient, however, must be watched constantly and guarded from carrying out activities that might be dangerous to himself and others. The acting-out, possibly psychotic patient must also be protected. It may be necessary to consider placement for these patients because the strong surveillance they need for their own protection and that of others may be otherwise impossible to achieve.

The aphasic patient who does not have these additional problems is perfectly trustworthy. He might not be able to take care of himself because of paralysis. It might be dangerous to leave him alone in a house, not only because of the muscular handicap but because his language disability prevents him from using the telephone to summon help. But these problems do not imply that he is intellectually impaired.

Should Others Do Things for the Brain Injured Person That He Can Do for Himself?

It is of the utmost importance that anything the patient is capable of doing safely, he must do alone or with minimal help and then, only when the help is really needed. There are many reasons for this and all of them for the patient's benefit. The only reason to do things for him that he can do or learn to do for himself is to make the doer feel better . . . because it saves time . . . or prevents a mess . . . or soothes guilt feelings . . . or is mistakenly attributed to lovingness or duty.

Sometimes, of course, saving time or preventing a mess are high priority items in a busy household. When this is so, it is perhaps good to take the short cut and give more help than usual, but if this becomes the standard procedure the patient is being harmed both physically and psychologically.

Weak muscles need exercise to become stronger. Unused muscles tend to atrophy or become weaker. To train a group of muscles to take over the function of paralyzed muscles requires much repetition of that action or series of actions. For example, a right-handed person who develops right hemiplegia must learn to eat, bathe, shave, brush his teeth, dress, comb his hair, and so on, with his left hand. One-handed dressing is very difficult. One has only to try it oneself with the non-dominant hand to realize the difficulties. It can be done but it requires much practice, especially with certain types of clothing. If the patient is not allowed to practice these new skills often and regularly, he will never master them. And he will not then gain the competence and self-esteem that each act of independence restores to him. Brain damage with resultant loss of muscular and communication skills produces a serious loss of self-esteem. Every situation that requires dependency where the patient was formerly independent increases this loss. There are many areas where he realistically must remain dependent; therefore, it is vital to assure that he learn to perform those skills possible for him to master.

The most efficient way to determine what the patient can be expected to accomplish is to have him evaluated by a rehabilitation team. This team usually includes a physician who is either an orthopedic surgeon, a physiatrist, or a neurologist, a physical and occupational therapist, and a speech pathologist. A vocational rehabilitation counselor and psychologist are usually available also, as well as a psychiatrist if mental competence is questionable. Many brain injured patients who do not have access to such a team never learn to walk again, to become toilet trained, or to communicate at a much higher level—even though they have the potential to acquire these skills—simply because no one realized they were capable of reaching these levels with training. Very often, even several years after onset, a family learns of a rehabilitation team and brings the patient for an evaluation. Countless patients and families in this position have learned to their great relief that the patient could be trained to reach much higher levels of functioning. This is not true of all brain damaged people, but thorough examination by a group of professionals can determine what he can and cannot be expected to do.

There are many devices and appliances available that assist hemiplegic and quadriplegic patients to become self-sufficient in a variety of situations (see Chapter XII). Even with a multitude of aids, however, a brain injured person is usually slower in performing many of the daily, necessary acts than he would be if someone helped him. Family members need to train themselves to accommodate for this. Because many patients have a poor sense of time, someone should arrange that he starts early enough to accomplish alone what has to be done. It may be necessary to check his progress from time to time, to be certain that he did not reach what is to him an insurmountable difficulty, but otherwise, he should be left alone to accomplish what it is known he can do if given ample time in which to do it.

Chapter III

General Information About Aphasia

What Is Aphasia?
Does Aphasia Improve or Completely Clear Up?
How Much Language Recovery Can Stroke Patients
Achieve?
How Much Language Recovery Can Brain Tumor Patients
Achieve?
How Much Language Recovery Can Head Injury or Brain
Disease Patients Achieve?
Why Is an Aphasic Patient So Inconsistent in Use of
Language?
Should He Be Told He Has Aphasia and That He Will
Recover Completely?
Is a Speech Pathologist Always Necessary to Treat
Aphasia?
Should Family Members or Friends Attend Speech
Therapy Sessions?
Should an Aphasic Be Permitted to Drive?
What Is a Stroke Club and How Can It Help Aphasic
Patients and Their Families?

What Is Aphasia?

Aphasia is the language disturbance caused by an injury to the language centers of the brain. In most of us these centers are in the left hemisphere. Aphasia means that losses have occurred in any or all of the ways involving *language* that we human beings use to communicate with one another. Not the mechanical, muscular means we utilize to express our language, because aphasia is *not* a muscular problem, but language itself. Aphasia includes the following language areas:

1. Understanding the speech of others
2. Speaking
3. Reading
4. Writing
5. Using gestures that are understandable to others
6. Understanding the gestures of others
7. Arithmetic

We might even include facial expressions, body language, and other more subtle methods of communication, but although these are all types of language, they have not been studied enough in relation to brain damage to be included here meaningfully.

Although aphasia can be so limited that only one language area of the seven listed above is affected, it is more usual for several or even all of them to have problems, especially in the early weeks following onset.

Does Aphasia Improve or Completely Clear Up?

Most aphasia improves. However, only a small percentage of aphasics will completely recover with no evidence that aphasia ever existed. These are generally the patients who displayed little loss by one month after the onset of a stroke. The course of improvement differs depending upon the cause of the condition. Aphasia caused by stroke will have a very different recovery rate from that produced by a head injury, a brain tumor, or brain disease; and these latter three will all differ from each other. Even among stroke patients, aphasia caused by a brain hemorrhage recovers at a different rate during the early months from that caused by thrombosis or embolism.

In addition to the cause of aphasia, the extent of brain damage and which additional parts of the brain suffer damage are important determinants in the ultimate potential for recovery. The physical, mental, and emotional well-being of the patient all play important roles in the rate and extent of his improvement. Good physical condition, a warm, loving, communicating environment, and relative freedom from stress can all contribute mightily to helping the patient reach his potential level of recovery. On the other hand, illness of any kind can interfere with improvement. Even a cold can cause a regression, although mild illnesses are apt to cause only temporary setbacks. The aphasic who is living in an emotionally disturbing environment will not be apt to improve as much as he is capable of improving. Brain injury that produces dementia or psychosis as well as aphasia will prevent language from improving; however, language therapy sometimes helps eliminate these conditions.

When there is extensive paralysis along with aphasia, the patient must struggle to learn how to handle his body in new ways. If he does not receive physical and occupational therapy during the early weeks after onset, he may develop contractures of certain muscles that will distort portions of his body permanently. Pain is another factor. Paralyzed limbs may be painful, severely so! Sometimes only surgery can provide release from this pain. These conditions interfere with smooth recovery of potential language.

The most positive factor in helping the aphasic reach his potential, aside from speech and language therapy, is to be in an environment that provides a great deal of communication experience. A patient whose only contact with others is to have his physical needs met—food, medication, rest, and cleanliness—but is left alone the rest of the time, will generally regress in language. Even a television set is better than no input at all, but it cannot replace live communication that includes the patient. Even if he understands little of what is said to him, it is important that he is spoken to and made to feel part of the group.

How Much Language Recovery Can Stroke Patients Achieve?

For aphasia caused by thrombosis or embolism, it is possible to predict what the language level will be at six months after onset by means of a particular test of aphasia (Porch, 1967) administered to the patient one month after onset. In order for the predicted level to be reached, it is necessary that recovery during that six-month period proceed without incident such as illness, chronic emotional distress, or dementia, and that another stroke does not occur. These conditions not only interfere with a patient's ability to reach his six-month potential for language improvement but also produce regression. This test must be given by a speech pathologist who has been specially trained to administer, score and interpret the test results; not all speech pathologists have had this training. Other aphasia tests are good for various reasons, but at this time I know of no other aphasia test that can give the specific prognostic information of where a patient's language level can be expected to reach in six months.

The first six months are a critical period. The aphasic who has been given good care will make what is called *spontaneous improvement* during this time. This is due to certain healing processes that take place in the brain and seem to reach their limit by six months after the CVA occurred. A few studies have found some language processes continue to improve spontaneously until nine months after onset, but that is generally considered the outside limit. The only exceptions I have ever encountered were when patients were prevented from making the early spontaneous recovery because of illness or poor care. Much later, when placed in a better environment with restored health, they made remarkable spontaneous improvement in language.

If the test results indicate that by six months after his stroke, or sooner, he should recover language well enough to return to work, plans made for the future will be entirely different from those where the prognosis indicates that there is no possibility for him to resume former responsibilities. Physically a patient may be fine, with no paralysis or weakness, but his language may be so impaired that returning to his former work will never be possible, although some people may be able to participate in a sheltered workshop.

The first aphasia test is best administered at one month after the CVA, not sooner, because during the first month language ability often changes rapidly. Treating aphasia during this period can be wasteful of time and money, except to provide emotional support which can be very important for some patients. At one time, earlier treatment was considered important. If there is *apraxia of speech* along with the aphasia, this should be treated as soon as the physician feels the patient is ready to receive therapy (see Chapter X).

The aphasic patient whose stroke was caused by hemorrhage, but who has not suffered widespread devastating brain damage, will generally improve in language much faster than the thrombo-embolic patient during the first two or three months. Because of this rapid improvement, test results during this period cannot be used to predict the level of language ability at six months. If the test is given monthly, which is the most desirable procedure, there will come a period when the early rapid improvement levels off. The patient will then follow the same course of recovery as if he had a thrombo-embolic stroke. This usually happens by the third or fourth month. At that time it becomes possible to predict the anticipated level at six months post onset.

At six months, nine at the most, stroke patients tend to plateau in language ability and usually remain at that level the rest of their lives, some even regressing, unless they receive language therapy or have contact with people who provide the correct kind of language stimulation suitable for their particular needs. With appropriate stimulation many aphasics can continue to progress for months and even years after the period of spontaneous recovery has been completed (Broida, 1977). This does not imply that their language skills will reach the level of their pre-stroke ability; but when communication is impaired, any improvement in one's capacity to exchange information with others vastly improves the quality of life.

The same test given at periodic checkpoints makes it possible to ascertain new potential goals and even to determine when no further improvement can be expected and, therefore, terminate treatment. For some this will be during the first year. For others, several or more years later.

How Much Language Recovery Can Brain Tumor Patients Achieve?

A brain tumor , whether benign or malignant, will naturally produce more problems as its grows in size. If the language areas are involved, language will become increasingly impaired. Speech therapy cannot help at this time. After the tumor is removed surgically or treated with radiation, language recovery will depend upon the amount of residual damage produced by the tumor and the surgery. Each person must be evaluated individually. Language therapy may then be of help to many patients in retrieving and reorganizing communication ability. Testing can sometimes indicate the next language level possible for the patient to attain and when to terminate treatment, but no ultimate goals in terms of months can be determined as is possible with the stroke patient.

How Much Language Recovery Can Head Injury or Brain Disease Patients Achieve?

Aphasia produced by head injury or disease such as Herpes Encephalitis follows unpredictable paths toward improvement. Often both hemispheres of the brain receive some injury in the accident or illness, so improvement depends upon the extent of the damage and what functions are impaired along with the language areas. Recovery, when it occurs, seems to come in periods of time following plateaus. These plateaus may last days, weeks, or even years. It does sometimes happen that many years after the injury aphasia will improve, especially if something occurs to improve the life-style of the patient.

At this time we have no way to predict the potential for language recovery in the patient whose aphasia was caused by a head injury or disease. The test results discussed in the two previous sections contain indicators that tell us what might be a goal for the next stage of improvement, but when the head injured patient reaches a plateau lasting several months, this does not necessarily mean he cannot improve further, as it usually does for stroke and tumor patients. When there is bilateral brain damage, however, even if the language becomes better integrated, the other disabilities may well prevent this patient from resuming former responsibilities.

Why Is an Aphasic Patient So Inconsistent in Use of Language?

At one moment he can say a word and respond appropriately to what is said to him. The next moment he cannot produce the word because he does not recall what it is, nor can he comprehend any words spoken to him. This is a maddening characteristic of many cases of aphasia. We all experience aphasic-like lapses when we attempt to recall a very familiar word or name that seems to be on the "tip of the tongue" but will not materialize. Hours later, when we no longer need it, it will suddenly "pop" into mind. So with the aphasic who tries with growing desperation to produce the word "water" when he is thirsty and, either nothing will come out, or a completely different, unwanted word like "shoe" might keep invading instead. Then, sometime later, when he no longer wants it, the word "water" will emerge, and even continue to emerge, when he is trying to say "sleep" or "hurt" or something else of great importance to him. The frustration for both the patient and listener is enormous. At one time the aphasic understands something long and complex that is said to him and a short time later he will not respond to a simple request such as "Open your mouth."

What causes this and how should others respond to it? Since it happens to all of us, although normally in isolated, widely spaced episodes, it is obviously a way our brains are capable of functioning under certain circumstances. There are neurophysiological explanations, but it is not within the scope of this book to deal with these aspects. One important fact that it reveals to us about the patient is that if at times he knows the meaning of a word such as "water," then he has not lost it entirely. It is there, stored in his brain, and it is now a question of finding ways to retrieve it dependably whenever he wants to use it. That is one of the important functions of language therapy, to help retrieve language processes that appear to be "blocked."

Aphasia may be likened to faulty wiring connected to a light bulb. The electric current may flow well for a period and then flicker on and off intermittently. Thus the aphasic may follow your instructions to close his eyes, but later stare at you blankly when you say the same thing, or open his mouth instead, or do something else inappropriate. Fatigue, tension, emotional upset, disturbed sleep, fear, happiness, pain, excitement—all of these can play a part in day to day fluctuations of language performance in aphasia. But even without any undue pressures, negative or positive, aphasia in many patients can fluctuate from moment to moment and day to day. Yet there is an overall consistency in aphasia in any one person so that the language pattern and level of performance can be adequately measured through testing, and progress, regression and plateaus can in general be reliably noted.

There is no correct way to respond to every instance of these inconsistencies. There is certainly one quite incorrect way and that is to insist that he certainly does know the meaning of the words or knows how to say what he wants, because he just knew them a short time ago. It is unnecessary, even undesirable, to remain in the language situation where the aphasic lost the word or the meaning of something he knew earlier. As with normal blocking, by getting into a different situation, taking the pressure off, so to speak, the correct response will sometimes emerge. If the patient appears to be trying to say something urgently that he cannot produce, there are methods that may be helpful (see Chapter V).

It is necessary to understand that there is no surefire method of producing adequate communication with an aphasic patient. By realizing this, one can possibly spare oneself and the patient many agonizing hours of trying to communicate. It is best to remain calm when all efforts to understand are unproductive, and to say to him gently but firmly that it is hard not to be able to say what he wants, but later the words might come to him, and then go on to something else—diverting if possible—so that he does not have to spend time miserably aware of his failure.

Should He Be Told He Has Aphasia and that He Will Recover Completely?

It is important to tell him he has aphasia but not that he will be completely fine again. I have listened to countless people in despair pat their aphasic husband's or wife's hand and assure them that in a few weeks they would be as good as new (with a pleading glance at me to confirm it, as much to them as to their spouse). I can certainly empathize with their wish to give this kind of assurance, but it is a misguided effort. It is unfair and potentially damaging to make promises that cannot be delivered. When time goes by, if the expected recovery does not take place, the patient does not know what to believe or whom to trust, and it is very necessary that he place much confidence in the people around him. Alone as he is behind the communication barrier that his aphasia has produced, there are certain anchors that can be given to him to help sustain him through the hard months ahead. Trust is a big one.

Primarily, it is important that he feels he has a condition that someone knows something about. A condition with a name. The fact that it has a name implies that others have had it and that there is probably a known way to deal with it. Anyone who has had an illness with symptoms unknown to him may recall the relief experienced when the illness was identified by name, even if the condition was very serious. This is the relief an aphasic patient feels: to know this dreadful inability to communicate as before has a name and is known to professionals who can do something about it.

He needs to be told he has had a stroke or an accident or whatever caused the aphasia, and that he will improve with time. No promise of any particular amount of time. Moreover, he can be assured that ways will be found to help him. Speech therapy is the most efficient means of providing such help, but if circumstances prevent this solution, a careful study of this book can initiate family and friends into procedures that may be valuable.

Is a Speech Pathologist Always Necessary to Treat Aphasia?

The only way to assure that the aphasic is recovering language ability to the level of his potential is to consult a speech pathologist who has had training and experience with adult aphasia. This does not necessarily mean that ongoing speech and language therapy with a professional is the only way to deal with aphasia. If there are physical or financial obstacles, the former including the lack of a speech pathologist in the community, there are optimal times when testing and ongoing speech therpy should be considered and times when other alternatives can be utilized.

A critical consideration is that language stimulation is of the utmost importance to the patient in order to make certain that he will make the gains he is capable of making and will not regress after he has reached his potential level of recovery. The patient whose physical needs are met, but who has little opportunity for language interaction with someone, will generally not progress during the early months when he should be spontaneously improving. In fact, under conditions of language neglect he will very likely regress.

The next critical factor is *what kind* of language stimulation? Is talking to him enough? Regardless of whether he understands or not? Should he be forced to talk? Should his errors be corrected? Should he be made to read and write and calculate? Is there a right and wrong period for certain language areas to be stressed? Can he be harmed by pushing him to respond or by working with certain language skills prematurely?

During the last ten years, great strides have been made through research and new techniques in testing aphasia that have given the field of clinical aphasiology long needed answers to these and other questions. It has been learned that there *are* particular times when certain language areas should not be dealt with in therapy (perhaps never for some aphasics); when certain language areas should be stressed, but in particular ways if the effort is to be of value; and when testing of language status is necessary to determine what has been gained, what is lagging or even regressing, and where the next concentration should be placed. Trying to stimulate a language skill before a patient is ready for it may do actual harm because of the inevitable failure that will result.

It is due to these considerations that a consultation with a speech pathologist should be sought, periodically at least, if it is at all feasible. If not, then the later chapters of this book, each devoted to one aspect of language, will provide some guidance for a home program. This cannot replace the benefits to be gained from ongoing speech therapy with a professional. If a speech pathologist cannot be found in the immediate community of the patient, the American Speech and Hearing Association (see Appendix A) will provide names of members in the nearest location. Speech pathologists are not all trained and experienced to treat aphasic adults, so it is necessary to learn their qualifications before seeking an appointment.

The ideal program for an aphasic patient is examination by a speech pathologist as soon as the physician feels it is safe to do so. If apraxia of speech (Chapter X) is found along with aphasia, the therapist will probably want to start working witn that immediately. Formerly it was felt that aphasia therapy should begin as soon after onset as possible. That is now known to be unnecessary, although it may give the patient hope and support. Aphasia therapy need not begin until after the first aphasia test, which is best given at one month post onset. Apraxia therapy, however, should start as soon as the patient can tolerate treatment. Aphasia not only fluctuates widely during the first month in some patients, but often improves quickly, even from day to day, making it impossible to tell what aspects of language impairment need to be treated. By one month, test results for thrombo-embolic patients are usually reliable and therapy can be planned according to the findings. For hemorrhage patients it is more likely to be the second or third month before test results can be depended upon to guide treatment. Early treatment may be advisable for the patient's emotional well-being, but the family must understand the distinction.

During the first six months following the onset of aphasia due to stroke, the spontaneous recovery from aphasia will follow a rather predictable course if the patient's physical, mental, and emotional status remain stable and he receives good language stimulation. If he is severely damaged in all language areas at the start, his recovery potential will be small. If he has minimal damage originally, the chances of almost total recovery are excellent without any speech therapy. Since the majority of aphasic involvement falls somewhere between these two extremes, these are the cases that need to be helped to their optimal potential by professional consultation. The important decision to make is when therapy would be the most beneficial.

If there is a limited budget, a good plan might be for the speech pathologist to set up a home treatment program for the first six months, with testing at one month, three months, and six months to determine if progress is moving as anticipated. After six months the difference between minimal and maximal language improvement for most patients from then on depends on speech therapy. All too often patients who have started therapy several years after their stroke have never received any kind of treatment earlier. After a program of therapy even years after onset, many of these patients make enough gain in language to improve greatly the quality of their communication skills, and therefore the quality of their lives. The same thing can happen in many cases with ability to walk, to become continent of bowels and of urine, and to develop self-help skills, so that it can be stated with great assurance that every brain damaged patient should have the opportunity to be examined by a rehabilitation team early after onset in order to learn how to help him achieve all the recovery his condition will allow. Without treatment it is likely that he will not reach his potential in any of these areas, including language.

Treatment for aphasia due to causes other than stroke needs individual assessment rather than blanket guidelines. Much depends upon the extent and kind of additional brain injury that exists along with damage to the language areas, as well as the patient's potential for physical improvement.

Any condition that is producing rapidly increasing impairment in most cases implies that speech therapy cannot help, except possibly to provide emotional support. If the family understands the limitations and chooses to provide speech therapy for this patient, there is no reason not to undertake it, if the speech therapist feels that such support can be of help. For patients whose aphasia was caused by a head injury, treatment can be very helpful during certain periods of improvement, enhancing the returning ability to organize thought and language; but during prolonged periods of plateaus it is often best to discontinue treatment until signs of new growth are noted. Some patients, however, can be helped through these periods faster if speech therapy is not interrupted. The speech pathologist treating the patient must make this determination.

Should Family Members or Friends Attend Speech Therapy Sessions?

There are pros and cons to this question that should be considered. Some speech therapists feel that a family member, friend, nurse, and others in frequent contact with the patient should attend the sessions—individually, of course—whenever possible. Others prefer that they do not attend. Here are some of the aspects to consider before making a decision.

First and foremost is the patient's reaction. If he is obviously agitated or distracted by the visitor, it is best to decide against attendance, at least during that particular time period. Perhaps several weeks later it can be attempted again. I have had patients who watch their spouses closely to judge their reaction to each of their responses. These patients become inhibited and fearful and cannot possibly progress as well as those who are not this concerned with the effect of each performance. When the spouses of these patients do not attend, and the contrast in behavior is very apparent, it becomes necessary to postpone the spouses' visits until the patient gains more confidence and independence. Closed circuit television or two-way mirror windows are good substitutes, if available.

The main purpose of including others in the therapy sessions is to train these people to use effective techniques in their daily contacts with the aphasic. The few hours spent in therapy each week are a small percentage of the total time a person has available for communication. If others besides the speech therapist use good and consistent methods of language stimulation, and avoid using useless or even harmful measures, the aphasic has a far better chance of improving faster and reaching higher levels than if only the therapist uses these methods. By reinforcing the returning skills often during each day in the particular ways taught by the therapist, these language elements stand a better chance of becoming well entrenched sooner.

Without guidance and some training by a speech pathologist the likelihood of misjudging the aphasic's language competence is very strong, and the selection of material for stimulation can be inappropriate, too often causing unfortunate reactions in the patient—some even to withdraw from further communication. The following situation occurs often enough to present it here as an example of an unhappy choice by a well-meaning, but uninformed, family member.

Most aphasic patients are right-handed, but many have paralyzed right hands. They are unable to write and their speech is so poor that they cannot be understood very often. To the observer who has not received proper instruction, it seems obvious that the reason the patient cannot write is because his right hand is paralyzed and his left hand clumsy. Therefore, this relative or friend, with only the most loving of intentions, will select as a gift a typewriter or a spelling board for the aphasic to use, hopefully as a means of communicating to others what he cannot say. These same people also tend to select such offerings as scrabble games, thinking that spelling and word games can be helpful. The effect of these unfortunate selections on the aphasic patient can be quite traumatic. The aphasic cannot write, even with his left hand, because his problem is with linguistics, not with mechanics. He cannot write because he cannot spell, because he has lost the word itself graphically, because he cannot formulate a phrase or sentence with pencil, pen, typewriter or spelling board. In many cases he has lost the alphabetical letter also. To present this particular aphasic patient with a typewriter is to imply to him that he should be able to use it, and if he cannot he is in very bad shape indeed—much worse than others realized. This failure is a source of the potential emotional harm to the patient caused by incorrect selection of materials.

In many cases of aphasia, writing is the most damaged language area and the last to return, if it ever does. Writing will be discussed more fully in Chapter VII, but at this time it should be explained that writing is not presented to an aphasic patient in therapy—except for copying of words, letters, or numbers—until or unless he is far advanced in language and is ready for graphic work. Many never will be ready. The person who *can* use a typewriter or spelling board for communication when he cannot talk is not apt to be aphasic but instead has either severe apraxia of speech or severe dysarthria (Chapter XI). These problems are sometimes mistaken for aphasia by professionals other than speech pathologists. Since the treatment for each condition is very different, examination by a speech pathologist is necessary for diagnosis and decision for therapy.

Another frequent error made by eager but uninformed people is to try to get the aphasic to name objects around him long before he is ready to do this. At the right time in his progress this is a fine and proper thing to do. Attempted too soon it can result in frightening him off altogether from any speech attempts. At the very least it can do no good when that same time could be used doing things that can help.

In spite of the advantages to the patient whose family and friends become trained to help him, many speech therapists refuse to let others attend the sessions for very good reasons. After having many negative experiences with the behavior of visitors and the sad effect of this behavior upon patients, many have decided that the risk of unpleasant consequences outweighs the advantages of permitting attendance. Some of the behavior therapists have experienced includes the visitor's laughing at the patient's attempts, which can be very threatening to him; giving cues or "body English" to some of his efforts when cues are undesirable; making such statements as "You can say that! You just said it yesterday;" acting impatient, bored, or even dismayed with the patient's responses; discussion during therapy time of their own problems that have nothing to do with the patient. All these and more are disruptive of good therapy. Laughter, cues, and encouraging statements all have their proper place and time in therapy, but the quality and timing of the reactions discussed here result in their inappropriateness.

There are other reasons for non-attendance of therapy sessions by family. Some cannot attend because work, child care, or their own disability make it unfeasible, but sometimes solutions can be worked out. One working husband found that if I arranged to see his wife one day a week during his lunch hour he would be able to attend that particular session regularly, to his wife's subsequent advantage. A wife who hires a baby sitter occasionally so she may attend therapy sessions can become more knowledgeable of and helpful with her husband's language disorder. There are, of course, some married couples who cannot work well with each other and should not try.

If family or friends are included in the therapy sessions it is good for them to try some of the techniques in the presence of the therapist before using them at home. Many tasks seem very simple but they may be misunderstood by amateur therapists and carried out incorrectly away from the office. The purpose of each task must be understood. Attitude in presenting the material is important. A calm, lightly pleasant presentation, unhurried and unperturbed by the patient's errors, is very necessary to acquire. Home sessions should be kept short, even of only ten minutes' duration several times a day. The patient should never be pressured to participate, but if refusal becomes habitual the therapist needs to know this. It may be due to material being presented that is too difficult and therefore too threatening. The best therapy for aphasia deals with those areas where the patient is just beginning to make errors, not where he usually fails. It is easy to present material that is too difficult if this principle is not well understood.

Workbooks (Stryker, 1975) are available that may be of help to family members in planning activities for home treatment sessions. There is a very real danger, however, in using workbooks, in that the temptation to move from page to page through the book can be strong, although the material, if used that way, will prove to be inappropriate for the patient's needs. If, however, the purpose of a task selected from the book is well understood and it can be used along with materials suitable for the patient's level of language disability, a workbook can be a very valuable aid. It is good to ask the patient's speech pathologist for a recommendation. Some may prefer that only the material presented in therapy should be used at home, for very good reasons.

In addition to learning how to help improve language use and to avoid errors in techniques, there is another valuable result of attending therapy sessions. The observer is in a favorable position to note when an important new step has occurred in the aphasic's language behavior away from therapy, and to make the therapist aware of the occurrence. Without learning what is important to report, he may not realize the significance of the new behavior. When an aphasic suddenly does something in language that he was unable to do earlier, the therapist may want to alter treatment so that this new behavior can be nurtured, but if the new response does not take place during treatment time, he cannot know about it. I have often received this kind of help from nurses who attended some sessions of aphasic patients still hospitalized and suddenly observed the patient responding in a new way on the ward.

Should the Aphasic Be Permitted to Drive

An automobile is an exceedingly dangerous weapon, as everyone well knows. To use it safely the driver must not only know how to operate a car and all the rules of the road, but must have dependable, fast reflexes and good use of vision, with correction if needed. Automobiles can be modified to accommodate drivers who have lost arms and legs, even some quadriplegics and paraplegics whose injury was to their spinal cords. *But no modification can be made to a car to accommodate certain kinds of damage to the brain of the driver.*

This does not mean that all aphasic people must not drive. It does mean, however, that since aphasia is due to brain damage, a careful assessment must be made of the aphasic's reflexes, visual status, judgment, basic ability to handle a car, and memory of the rules. A hemiplegic is not in the same position as someone who has lost the use of one or even all four limbs for reasons other than brain damage. The brain injury may have reduced reaction time subtly, but just enough to produce a serious driving risk. It may have caused *visual field cuts* so that parts of the vision in each eye have been destroyed. This results in a serious driving hazard. This visual loss may be undetected and unrealized, even by the patient, because he is able to see. If he wears glasses he may be cleaning them often, thinking that something on the lens is interferring with his clear vision. He realizes a difference in how he sees, but cannot pinpoint where the difference lies. If he drives with these blind spots in his visual fields, a serious tragedy can result.

Aphasics who have no muscular impairment often feel they should be able to drive. Brain damage itself can impair judgment, especially if the right hemisphere is affected, but even without this additional damage, the brain injured person is not in a position to decide his competence to drive.

For many reasons, it is harder for wives to refuse to let their husbands drive than for husbands to keep their wives from driving when it appears evident that they present driving hazards. Wives who never drove or whose husbands have been the decision makers for the family have particular difficulty. Driving is an ego-involving issue for many men. When an insecure wife finds herself in this sensitive position of prohibiting the driving of an aphasic husband who is determined to drive, she may find it impossible to stand up to him, short of selling the car and thereby facing his everlasting wrath. Many wives have told me tearfully of finding their husbands tearing apart every drawer in the house looking for the car keys they have hidden.

In some communities there are centers, often connected with a large rehabilitation clinic, where the driving ability of people who have suffered brain damage can be tested. All potential problem areas are carefully checked, and anyone likely to pose a driving risk is denied a license to drive. If the test determines that the aphasic must not drive because he cannot react reliably under stress situations, the wife has a strong ally to support her refusal, although this does not always help.

Lack of ability to read does not stand in the way of getting a driver's license, since many people cannot read the language of the country through which they are traveling. This is why international symbols are used on roads and highways all over the world. But these symbols are a form of language, and many aphasics cannot understand these any better than they can understand the printed word. Not comprehending critical symbols can cause serious accidents.

There is no easy solution to a situation where driving must be denied someone who insists upon driving. The very fact of the insistence, in the face of evidence that driving is hazardous for this person, provides further conformation of poor judgment. But the refusal must be firm, and all possible support for the position should be sought.

What Is a Stroke Club and How Can It Help Aphasic Patients and Their Families?

A Stroke Club, or Resocialization Club as it is sometimes called, is composed of brain injured people and their families, who meet weekly or biweekly for several important purposes, some social, some supportive, and some to dispense information.

People whose life-styles have been altered drastically due to physical and communication limitations following brain damage often discover that it is difficult or even impossible to continue relationships with their old friends and associates. This not only refers to the patients but most certainly to their spouses also. Wives and husbands may find that after the aphasic's physical condition stabilizes and the new status is finally realized by all, adjustments in old relationships have to be made. Those fortunate people who are surrounded by large families and a life-long accumulation of friends, all of whom are devoted and able to accept the altered conditions, may not need to investigate Stroke Clubs as an important resource for themselves, although even they may obtain some invaluable information when attending the meetings. But many people these days have moved to new communities where they have not had time to acquire friends at the level of devotion that can survive the changes brain damage may cause. It is for these people that Stroke Clubs provide the most value.

Spouses of aphasic people may become intensely lonely. Their marital companion can no longer communicate as before. Their relationship has been forced to change in many ways with necessary shifts in responsibilities and dependency. Old friends do not always include them as before and, as time goes on, this becomes more and more obvious. Bitterness, anger, and feelings of rejection can become overwhelming, and added to these come very understandable feelings of being trapped, which may lead to guilt feelings and depression.

At various times during our lives we all must come to the realization that some friendships are based entirely on certain mutuality of needs and interests, and when these needs and interests change for any reason, the basis for a particular friendship no longer exists. The strain involved in trying to continue a relationship that no longer contains enough nurturance to sustain it becomes apparent, and after a while one or the other discontinues the effort.

It is certainly rough for the family members who find themselves in this position—deserted and trapped, with no apparent recourse; but, after all, what else can bowling buddies, bridge or square dance partners, or conversation communicants do when one half of a couple can no longer bowl or play bridge or dance or communicate?

Probably the most helpful message to convey to the lonely mates is that this is where they can make a very important decision that may well affect the rest of their lives. They can *decide* to remain lonely and depressed and bitter and trapped; or they can *decide* to find new friends with whom to share their new life style and interests. This is the main purpose of the Stroke or Resocialization Clubs: to provide an environment where people can come together who share a specific problem—a family member who has suffered brain injury. Not only can they use guest speakers or whatever expertise they may have developed themselves to share with each other solutions to common problems, but they also have an opportunity to find a rich new source of friends. Even if only one couple is found in this club with whom a family can establish a close relationship, the enrichment of life for both couples is strong.

In addition to a resource for new friendships, the Stroke Club provides an environment where the aphasic and wife or husband can feel less isolated by being with people who share their problem. They can plan activities where all can participate: pot luck dinners, bus trips to places of interest, bowling leagues, lectures, discussion groups on topics of shared concern, movies, theatre groups, even travel to distant places—the list is endless. Parents, children, and close friends of the patient are eagerly urged to attend also. Those people who have suffered brain injury but have no family or friends to attend with them should be encouraged to attend alone. Arrangements can often be made to have them picked up by other members and made to feel welcome when they arrive.

When a community has not yet organized a Stroke Club and there is no local group such as the American Heart Association (Appendix A) to help one get started, interested professionals or family members should contact the national headquarters of the Heart Association for suggestions on how to procede. Getting in touch with other families who might be interested can be done through the nearest rehabilitation center, speech pathologists, occupational and physical therapists, and physicians. These clubs usually grow so fast once started that they often have to split into smaller neighborhood or interest groups, which demonstrates the urgent need for them and the reception that efforts to organize such a group will be apt to receive.

Chapter IV

Aphasia: Understanding the Speech of Others

Is It Possible to Be Certain That an Aphasic Understands What Is Said to Him?

Can His Poor Understanding Be Due to a Hearing Loss?

Do All Aphasic Patients Have Difficulty Understanding Speech?

Are There Degrees of Difficulty Among Aphasics in Understanding Speech?

If He Is Bilingual Does He Understand Better in One Language Than in Another?

How Can He Be Helped to Understand What Is Said to Him?

Is It Possible to Be Certain That an Aphasic Understands What Is Said to Him?

Probably one of the greatest shocks to the family and to many paramedicals who work with an aphasic is to learn that he does not understand a great deal of what is said to him and around him when they have been under the impression that he understands well. The majority of people with aphasia have some reduction in their ability to understand the speech of others. Amazingly, even those with a severe inability to understand are often believed to understand well by those close to them. How can this happen?

Many aphasics become very adept at noting gestures, facial expressions, eye movements, and the body language of others. Therefore, when these are used along with speech, the patient responds to them correctly often enough to lead the speaker to believe it was the words themselves to which he was responding. In many cases, some of the words do carry meaning to the patient, especially if used along with all the other cues. Anyone who has ever tried to communicate with a person who did not speak his language but whose language he understood slightly, will realize how helpful all these accompanying gestures can be in conveying meaning. When verbal language fails to communicate meaning we all use every other avenue possible to try to comprehend when it is important to do so. Aphasics often become very sensitive to situations, to time of day, and other cues. Thus, if a nurse comes in at a time when she normally gives him a backrub and says, "Turn over," accompanying these words with a flip of her hand, and he then turns over, she will report that he understands her speech well. If, however, he is given the same instructions at another time of day, perhaps by someone who would not be expected to give a backrub, and with no accompanying gesture, not even of the head, nor with any telltale eye movement, he may look at the speaker in bewilderment indicating complete lack of understanding.

Many aphasics who understand poorly and have little or no ability to speak develop a habit of nodding "yes" and even smiling as if in agreement with everything said to them. The conversation can go something like this: "Are you feeling good today?" Smile-nod. "Do you want to go home?" Smile-nod. "Do you want me to stay and visit with you?" Smile-nod. The questioner will be positive that the patient understood his words well. Perhaps he did, but the only way to be certain is to reword the questions so that the patient will have to give a different response to mean the same thing. For example: "Do you feel bad today?" Smile-nod. "Do you want to stay in the hospital?" Smile-nod. "Do you want me to leave you alone here now?" Smile-nod. Demonstrations like this are often needed to convince others of the patient's poor understanding of speech.

For many reasons, it is very important for those who deal with the patient to know how little he understands. Some aphasic patients are considered difficult to deal with when the real trouble is their poor comprehension of what was said to them by people who did not realize they could not understand well. I know an aphasic patient who was put out of a nursing home because he insisted on smoking in his room after being told repeatedly that it was against the fire laws for him to do this. Only after his comprehension was tested and it was learned how little he understood of the spoken and written word did the owners of the home realize how badly they had judged and treated him. Yet he was so animated in his responses that everyone thought he fully understood their words and the printed "No Smoking" signs.

When important decisions must be reached and the aphasic's ability to understand has been misjudged, serious errors may be made in carrying out what is believed to be his intent. If his limitations in comprehension are fully understood, yet his concurrence is needed for some legal, economic, or otherwise important step, care will be taken to use necessary precautions, either by postponing the decision until his comprehension improves (if it will), or by taking other steps.

Why do some aphasics "pretend" to understand when they do not? Some find it humiliating and frightening to be in this position. Everyone around them seems to be talking in a foreign tongue. When nodding and smiling gets some kind of positive results, they continue to use this technique if only to gain time, perhaps hoping that all will become clarified and they will understand without betraying themselves to the others. Other aphasics may do this because they are weakened and do not want to cope. If nodding and smiling gets people off their backs for a while, they will use this response repeatedly.

There are many different ways an aphasic patient can misunderstand what is said to him. Some understand only verbs and seem to have lost all the nouns. Others have lost all the so-called "little words," such as "the," "and," and all the prepositions. Some will understand fairly well if simple sentences are used with only one message unit per sentence, but totally misunderstand everything if complex sentences are spoken with two or more messages. Examples are probably the best way of describing the ways various patients can be understanding what they hear. Let us suppose that what is said is: "I made some fresh coffee. Would you like a cup?" Here are some of the ways he may interpret what is said depending upon his particular kind of comprehension problem:

1. GARSHASH SNOOP OONUP.

Total jargon with no inkling of any meaning.

2. COFFEE.

He understands the first noun; everything else is meaningless and becomes an overload, so that the second noun, "cup," is also lost. In this case a nod would be valid if he wants a cup of coffee and it would not be realized that he understood only one word out of the eleven uttered.

3. CUP.

Only the last noun has meaning, because nouns are all he understands and his memory cannot retain the first noun by the time the second one is spoken. With only the word "cup" he might not have enough information to reply properly to the question. If cup reminds him of tea and he gets coffee, there might be repercussions.

4. _____ COFFEE _____ CUP.

He understands the nouns and probably can respond correctly with this much information. It would not be realized that he missed the meaning of nine other words.

5.   MADE   TEA.   LIKE   SAUCER?

He understands the verbs but confuses the nouns for other nouns with closely associated meanings. If he dislikes tea and responds according to his understanding of what was said, and then saw the questioner drinking coffee later without offering him any, his reaction might be of anger. "Saucer" may have puzzled him, but it was in the ballpark.

6.   MADE   SLEEVES   LIKE   ROBIN?

He again understands the verbs but completely misunderstands the nouns so that the entire message is meaningless.

7. I MADE US   FEEFUS. WOULD YOU LIKE BROOPER?

Jargon is interspersed with meaning but not enough to inform him of the intent.

8. He repeats perfectly the entire series of words spoken to him, perhaps even several times, as if by repeating it he will understand it, but it remains totally meaningless. This is perhaps one of the most difficult kinds of comprehension problems to grasp. He obviously has no difficulty receiving the words correctly and retaining them, even in the correct order, but they make no sense at all to him.

It should be obvious that understanding of speech is a very complex function and can become defective in many ways that may easily be misunderstood if others are not aware of the possibilities. Even in this presentation only a few of many kinds of difficulties in comprehension have been discussed. As language becomes more complex and abstract, problems multiply. People who understand well at one level may become totally lost at a higher level of language usage.

When more than one person is talking, the aphasic who understands well in a one-to-one situation may lose all ability to follow what is being said. He may then refuse to attend any group functions, as any of us would if we could not follow the conversation. I have heard these kinds of patients described as anti-social, as others try to force them to attend groups that are felt to be good for them. The isolation an aphasic feels in a group where he cannot understand what is being said needs to be recognized by others. If this same person can understand better when with only a few people who try hard to include him in the conversation, perhaps a small group within the larger one can be organized so that the aphasic can attend the function but feel more secure.

Can His Poor Understanding Be Due to a Hearing Loss?

If he had a hearing loss before the onset of aphasia there is no doubt that this loss contributes significantly to his difficulty in understanding speech. But hearing loss and inability to understand the speech of others are two entirely different problems. If one does not understand Greek, it will not be understood any better if it is shouted loudly. If, however, one understands a little Greek it is important that it be heard very clearly so that those words that may have meaning come through quite distinctly. The words must not be masked by other noises, such as the rumble of several voices talking at the same time, as at a cocktail party. If one wears a hearing aid, it must be functioning well at all times.

It is unlikely that a stroke will produce a hearing loss or further impair an existing loss. A tumor may produce a hearing loss, depending on its location. Brain injury due to an accident may include damage to the auditory nerve resulting in hearing impairment. But a distinction must be made between reduced ability to understand speech due to a hearing loss and that due to aphasia. In hearing loss some or all of the sounds that go into the ear cannot be carried to the brain for interpretation because something is blocking their way. In aphasia, the sounds are transmitted, fully intact, to the center in the brain that decodes the messages they carry, but the decoder is damaged. That, in great oversimplification, is the essence of the aphasic's difficulty understanding speech. Obviously, if impaired sounds due to a hearing loss are carried to an impaired decoding system, the entire process is further marred; therefore, it is important to know if a hearing loss exists along with the aphasia. When there is a question, an audiometric test should be given, but only by someone who understands the limitations of aphasia so the tests can be modified accordingly. All people who test hearing are not trained to understand aphasia well enough to test an aphasic validly.

Do All Aphasic Patients Have Difficulty Understanding Speech?

Most do, especially during the early period after onset of aphasia. Physicians usually speak of it as being either *receptive aphasia*, in which understanding of speech and reading are the recognized problems (language a person receives), *expressive aphasia*, in which speaking and writing are the problems (language a person uses to express himself), or *receptive-expressive aphasia* which is a combination of the two. Speech pathologists generally find that it is most often the combination condition in a variety of patterns that they encounter in treatment. It is unusual to find a purely receptive or purely expressive aphasic.

For any aphasic patient the safest assumption to make is that regardless of how well he seems to be understanding speech, there is a very good chance that he is experiencing some change in his ability to comprehend it. Whether his loss is very mild or very severe, the probability is strong that others may not be recognizing the problems he has. Sometimes, when the impairment is very mild, only a speech pathologist probing for difficulties in subtle, complex, and abstract language comprehension and measuring his auditory retention span, can detect the problem.

Are There Degrees of Difficulties Among Aphasics in Understanding Speech?

Degrees of difficulties in understanding speech cover a wide range, from extremely mild so that only the aphasic knows that he has experienced a change, through all manner of increasing impairment, to total inability to understand anything said at any time.

A very mild difficulty may manifest itself in one way only and that is in his need to take a bit more time than he formerly required to assimilate things said to him and fully understand them. We all have this difficulty normally at times, either because we are tired or distracted or because the material coming at us is somewhat complex or more difficult than our level of knowledge of the subject permits us to cope with easily. Given extra time to process the incoming information, we may eventually absorb and understand. Although not always. This need for extra *processing time* is a frequent characteristic of aphasia. In mild difficulties it is often the only manifestation.

Even the most mildly impaired aphasic has varying thresholds, so that if he is fatigued, overstimulated, unusually concerned or tense, and if someone is speaking to him very fast or with too many details at that particular time, he may reach an overload and fail to understand the real meaning of what was said no matter how much processing time he takes.

For these reasons it is always a good idea to allow an aphasic extra time to respond to what is said, to slow one's rate of speech (especially if one tends to talk fast), and to avoid presenting too many details in one group of sentences.

Another difficulty aphasics may have is not understanding speech until the statement is repeated or even rephrased. Some patients require repetitions of 50 percent or more of everything said to them, others only as little as 10 percent or even less. Some need a cue such as a key word repeated, before they can tune in to what is being discussed. If time is taken to set the stage, so to speak, they may follow with better comprehension.

Aphasics with impairments of auditory retention span (Chapter II) may only understand when short phrases containing only one unit of information per phrase are used. For this patient the information or questions put to him must be presented in individual units. Thus, instead of saying "Aunt Mary is in town. Shall we drive over and visit her at Jerry's house?," the message might be stated something like this: "Aunt Mary. Remember Aunt Mary?" When it is certain he knows who is being discussed, by repeating if necessary, add: "She is staying with Jerry." This must be digested and understood before asking: "Do you want to visit her?"

Some aphasics confuse similar objects. The word "spoon" is said and he thinks of it as "fork." Someone says "dollar" and he perceives it as "quarter." If a plane trip is discussed he may be thinking train or automobile.

Those patients who understand no nouns will have great difficulty following what is said to them no matter how carefully it is delivered. If they understand the nouns but have few verbs and no prepositions, they will know what the subject is that is being discussed but not what is said about it. Understanding parts of speech is not an all-or-nothing matter. He may understand 25 percent or 75 percent of nouns and 10 percent or 30 percent of verbs. These are not necessarily the same ones each time they are spoken to him.

There are aphasics who seem to misunderstand completely everything said to them. If you tell them to point to the telephone, they may pick up a book. There are those who may make mistakes on their first try, but then hear the words reverberating and realize they have made an error and hasten to correct it if they can. An aphasic who is able to correct his errors without someone's intervention is at a higher level than one who either does not realize his errors or who shrugs helplessly, unable to correct them. In fact, when a patient who has been functioning in the latter categories suddenly self-corrects an error, this is viewed by speech pathologists as an important sign of progress.

Some aphasics watch the speaker but make no move to indicate they understood what was said. Among these are people who understand so little and are so fearful of making a wrong response that they do not try, even though they may tune in to a word here and there correctly. At this same level of poor understanding are many of those who nod and smile at the speaker although they really have understood little that was said.

At the lowest level of comprehension difficulties are those who do not even seem aware that someone is trying to speak to them. These are very severely impaired patients. If this condition exists in a thrombo-embolic stroke patient by one month post-onset, prognosis is very poor. Other causes of aphasia, however, may present a different prognosis for a patient in this condition, so each must be discussed with the physician.

I have used the words "tuned in" several times when describing auditory comprehension. It is a phrase very descriptive of what happens to many aphasics. Some have patterns of comprehension in which they have difficulty at the start, when a new subject is introduced. After an early series of errors they "tune in" and then follow well whatever is said. Others start off well but seem to fatigue and lose ability to remain "tuned in." But most seem to fade in and out wthout any particular pattern. The important thing is for the speaker to realize that these patterns can very likely be occurring, and that his understanding of what is said is not an all-or-nothing situation. Because he understands well at one moment does not guarantee that what follows will be understood at all.

If He Is Bilingual, Does He Understand Better in One Language than in Another?

Although some speech pathologists have reported that the original language (mother tongue) of the aphasic usually returns first, I have never found this to be true, nor have any of the colleagues I have questioned about this. It has been my experience that wherever we could actually check the status of both languages, difficulty was about equal. One of the misleading aspects that leads some people to believe there is greater competence in the mother tongue when it is a different language from English, is the intact presence of the melody and accents of the original language. For example, take the case of an aphasic whose native tongue was Spanish and who retained his Spanish accent although he became fluent in English. People treating him did not understand Spanish, so his utterances, which were total jargon in both languages, sounded to them as if they were Spanish because of the melody and accents associated by them with that language. This patient had difficulty understanding English, so they assumed that he understood Spanish better. Not until we found someone who knew Spanish well did we learn the truth. To take this further, if the family of such a patient speaks mostly, or even only, Spanish, they may have made the same error that other families make when judging the patient's ability to understand. If he is adept at understanding gestures and situations, they may believe he is understanding their words; therefore, when asked if he understands Spanish well, they can very well insist that he does.

Only by testing his ability in the same tasks in both languages can the true determination be made. One way to do this is to place about five objects in front of him. Indicate to him that he is to point to each one as it is named. This must be done in random order. Two people may be needed to carry this out if no one person speaks both languages equally well. If he has no difficulty with either language at this level, a more difficult task needs to be selected, such as asking him to point to the object used for reading, for drinking, etc. When it is clear that he understands what he is supposed to be doing and is responding to the best of his ability, add more objects so that there are about ten. The task should be repeated in both languages several times, not necessarily immediately, and his responses noted. If he follows the pattern that I have found, he will have about the same number of errors in both languages.

What should be done with this information? If he is to have speech therapy or if a home program is to be attempted, one language should be used in all his exposures as much as possible. If he is to live in an English speaking environment then that language should be English. Spontaneous recovery will probably occur in both languages at about the same rate, but therapy should push him well beyond that, and it is best done in the language that will be most important for him to use in the years ahead. If he is to live with his family who only speak Spanish and there is little likelihood that he will ever be able to return to work where English is used, then every effort should be made to have his therapy conducted in Spanish. Of course, if there is no choice, the language most readily available to the people who are helping him must be used.

How Can He Be Helped to Understand What Is Said to Him?

There are two aspects of this question, each handled differently from the other. The first has to do with times when it is very important for him to understand what is being said if it is at all possible. The second concerns techniques such as those used in therapy or in a home treatment program that are designed to improve his ability to understand speech.

When it is desirable that he understands what is being said, every possible means should be utilized along with speech to improve the chances that the meaning is coming through to him. This includes using gestures, facial expressions, eye movements, body language, pictures, and the written or printed word. Some aphasics who understand little speech are able to read some words, perhaps only nouns or verbs, that when used together with all the other cues will aid to get the meaning across. If the situation is important for him to understand, it is necessary to check his comprehension by rephrasing, to be doubly certain that he really understands. If, no matter how many aids are used, it is still clear that he does not really understand, it is best to give it up rather than continue until he is overcome with frustration and feelings of complete failure. In fact, if no attempt works, it is best to give him something to do that he can perform easily, so that he is left with positive feelings.

In therapy attempted in a home program, a totally different approach is required. This also applies to paramedicals, such as physical therapists, who might want to use some techniques for aiding comprehension while working on other things. To help improve the process of understanding speech, it is important to: (1) use speech alone, with no other gestural or written cues; (2)

work only at the level where he is just beginning to have difficulties, never beyond his capability of producing at least 80 percent correct responses on a selected task; (3) expect him to respond only through means that are not damaged; (4) try to use material that is important to him, of interest to him, never things that are outside of his experience or concern; (5) not take it for granted that because he understands something at one time that he now understands it all the time.

When working with him to improve comprehension of speech, it is necessary to omit all extraneous cues other than the spoken word itself and the object or picture that word represents. He might be asked to point to the door, the wheelchair, the light, the floor, the doctor, a picture of his wife, a cup, etc. It might be necessary to demonstrate what pointing means, but the noun itself should be represented only by the word he hears and the actual object or its picture. Use only two or three of these at a time until he gets them right often. If he cannot have any successes with them as nouns, he might have better understanding if they are described like this: "Point to the one used for drinking." If none of these work, then it is necessary to back up and only say the names of objects and people to him, expecting no response from him except attention. In a few weeks it might be good to try the first approach again, and if he has some successes, proceed with it slowly, not eliminating the naming technique. When he can point successfully to as many as ten objects during one session, it is good to change the task concerning these objects. For example, when he clearly knows the word "glass," instead of telling him to point to it, introduce something like "Pick up the glass," or "Give me the glass."

A session with one task may last as long as ten minutes, perhaps repeated several times a day if that is feasible. Never during these sessions when his auditory comprehension is the task at hand, should he be required to name the objects. Nor should he use any other defective language area, such as writing, to demonstrate that he knows what is being said. A gestural response is best, unless he has two paralyzed hands. In that case an undamaged response system must be utilized, such as looking at the correct object or nodding his head as someone else points, if it is certain that his nods can be trusted to mean "yes."

When there is doubt about his comprehension or it has not yet been checked, the best approach is merely naming objects to him. Everyone who comes in contact with him soon after onset can give him very valuable input by stating the names of things as he uses them. A nurse bringing him breakfast can name each dish as she puts it before him. Later she might ask him to pick up his orange juice, but at the start it is best for her only to name it.

There is an unfortunate tendency among many people in contact with aphasics to say to them, long before they are ready for this: "Tell me the name of this," or "What do you call this?" And the aphasic will stare at them forlornly unable to produce the name. If, instead, the request had been to point to that object, a meaningful step toward retrieving comprehension and the name itself would have been taken.

Using material that has significance to the patient is of the utmost importance. Pictures of family members are of first order importance, and these include beloved pets. Words like toilet, water, doctor, nurse, favorite foods, shower, bath, shave, sleep, bed, chair are all of everyday significance. Later it is wise to introduce words for the patient's special interests. There is a dramatic difference between the responses of patients to those items close to them emotionally and to items for which they have no special concern. A patient of mine had been a chef, but due to the circumstances of his hospitalization, no one knew this had been his occupation until many months after treatment started. He had become withdrawn and had definitely reached a plateau in language improvement, although test results indicated he had a higher ultimate potential. When I learned accidentally of his former vocation, I brought in cook books, pictures of pots and pans, and cooking utensils of many descriptions. He visibly perked up and months later was actually able to give me some simple, tasty recipes. It would never have occurred to me to use these particular items with a male patient, yet they were the only source of ego involvement and identity that could pull him out of his deep depression and give him an incentive to work harder. He made strong strides in the months that followed.

Another patient came into treatment each day showing his ID card identifying him as a Major in the army. By using pictures of different military ranks and other things related to army life, he was very inspired to work hard on his comprehension capability.

The amateur tends to move too fast through therapeutic steps. Many repetitions are required to be sure responses become well entrenched and easily retrieved. Just because a patient knows something one day does not guarantee that he will know it the following day or week. Fluctuations are common. This does not mean that every word must be painstakingly drilled. If that were true, speech therapy would not be possible. These techniques are used to try to awaken a process. If they are to succeed, the groundwork must be slow and careful. When the process is being revived successfully, a cluster of words not worked on begins to emerge and fall into place. Sometimes nouns, then verbs; later prepositions. When many needed kinds of words return, phrases start to become more meaningful, and finally sentences.

Not every aphasic can go through all the steps. Each has a limit to the amount of competence he may achieve and cannot be stretched beyond that limit. Therapy attempts must never jump from pointing to an object to carrying out three-part commands with no intervening steps. Only by progressing logically can the limits be determined when they are reached.

In addition to understanding the actual words, the patient's auditory retention span must be taken into account. He may well understand a one-unit brief sentence, spoken to him slowly and giving him ample time for response, but if two or more units are presented at one time he may lose it all. If he is asked "Do you want eggs?" and later "Do you want cereal?" he may fully comprehend and respond appropriately with yes to each or to one. But when asked "Do you want eggs or cereal?" he may stare blankly at the speaker. During therapy sessions these limits can be well established.

Chapter V

Aphasia: Speech Difficulties

Are There Different Patterns of Speech Problems in
Aphasia?

What Can Be Done About Aphasics Who Use Profanity
Liberally? Why Do They Do It?

Can It Help to Ask an Aphasic the Names of Things
Around Him?

How Can He Be Helped to Find the Word He Wants to
Say?

Should Faulty Pronunciation and Other Errors Be
Corrected?

Is It Wise to Pretend to Understand Him When He Is Not
Understood?

Is Singing of Any Value to Aphasics?

What Should Be Done When He Keeps Repeating the
Same Word Although Trying to Say Something
Else?

What Should Be Done When an Aphasic Cannot Say
Something He Said Well Earlier?

How Can Others Help Him to Communicate More
Easily?

What is a Communication Notebook and How Can It
Help?

Are There Different Patterns of Speech Problems in Aphasia?

The most obvious sign of aphasia is the disturbance in the patient's speech. He may have far more impairment in writing, reading, and comprehension than in speech, but to others his speech disability is the most noticeable difference. Aphasia usually produces a "word finding" problem, but there are various patterns of these problems depending upon the location and extent of the brain injury. Here are some of the ways different aphasic patients may try to say "Bring me a glass of water, please."

1. Doo doo doo. Doo doo doo.
2. Amen. Yes, amen.
3. Oh darn it. Oh, darn it. (Or stronger language.)
4. Affig shizl per duh fanzer.
5. Eekur uh-me uh-shass pass uh wating uh water-shess.
6. Bring me a ducher of shantow, please.
7. Bring me a desk of clocks, please.
8. Bring me a dish of milk, please.
9. Bring me-uh the -uh- pan- no uh the pan -no uh-oh, skip it. I know . . . the pan. Oh, no.
10. Bring uh-give -of, you know, what you eat, no, uh-drive, no drink -yes, that's it, drink, coffee, uh, no, clear stuff -uh. Yes.
11. Water.
12. Glass.
13. Drink.
14. Bringing her drinking.

Aphasic patients have difficulties with words, either with the word itself or the meaning of the word. They often lose whole categories of words such as nouns or verbs. Some aphasics have no trouble with these but have lost all the "little words"—the prepositions, conjunctions, and articles. Their speech then sounds like a telegraphic message with only key words used. In fact, this type of aphasic utterance is called *telegraphic* speech.

The aphasic is usually able to say a word or short phrase if he is given a model to imitate. He will not necessarily be able to reproduce it again a short time later without the model being repeated but he should have no trouble imitating unless he has a particular kind of aphasia called *fluent aphasia*, or he does not understand what is wanted of him or if he has the additional problems of apraxia of speech (Chapter X) or dysarthria (Chapter XI).

The *fluent aphasic* may talk a great deal, perhaps even incessantly, but he generally makes little sense. There are variations of fluent aphasia but all are based on an auditory problem in which the patient has trouble monitoring his own speech through his hearing. The words he thinks he is uttering are coming out all wrong but he is unaware of it. They may sound like pure jargon or like "double talk" in which there are real words used inappropriately or real words mixed with jargon so that the listener may at first believe the problem to be his own, that he missed something important in the outpouring. Melody and inflection are usually intact, giving further credence to the double-talk similarity. A stream of such utterances may end in inflections that indicate a question has been asked and the aphasic is awaiting a reply. Since the listener has no idea what he was asked, he can only shrug helplessly, hoping for a clue. Anger and frustration can be the result of such encounters. Explanations to the aphasic may be of little value as his auditory problem often includes poor understanding of the speech of others. What is amazing is that if the listener imitates the patient's jargon, he will be apt to look startled or to laugh at what he hears as pure nonsense, not having any realization that his own speech sounds this way. If a tape recording is made of his speech, his reaction will be the same, not connecting it at all with his own production.

The same injury that produced aphasia can also produce apraxia and dysarthria. If an aphasic patient is also apraxic, he is apt to have great difficulty imitating words or phrases, although he may be able to utter those words automatically at times. If he is dysarthric he will have paralysis or weakness of some muscles needed to produce certain speech sounds or even voice itself. It a patient has all three, or even two of these conditions, the problems of diagnosis and treatment are compounded, but it is necessary to distinguish among them whenever possible because treatment is very different for each.

"Automatic speech" is another phenomenon of aphasia that is extremely frustrating to many listeners as well as to the aphasic. Often it accompanies severe apraxia of speech. In automatic speech the aphasic may only be able to produce a repetitive group of sounds such as "dee dee dee" whenever he tries to say something, or repeat phrases such as "Nothing doing" every time he tries to talk. *Profanity* is a form of automatic speech. The next section will deal with this phenomenon that is so disturbing to many families and, at times, to hospital ward personnel.

Perseveration means to contribute the same action over and over when it is no longer appropriate. Some aphasics tend to perservate in speech so that when they respond with a word, which may or may not be appropriate, they seem unable to turn it off. They continue to produce that word with nearly every effort to speak for the next indefinite period of time. Some will struggle to break free of it and, finally succeeding, will fall into another "perseveration trap" with a different word a short time later. In the morning an aphasic may get stuck with the word "egg," so that he will say something like: "I want shave. Where is egg, I mean, uh- shave, uh- egg, no- face- egg, no- egg, uh- razor. Yes, razor." Then "razor" may become his perseverative utterance for the rest of that day or even week.

Great patience is required with an aphasic who works his way painfully through many detours, false starts, perseverations, and repetitions until he finally makes his thoughts known to the listener. This kind of aphasic has good self-monitoring ability so he can immediately recognize his incorrect effort, sometimes even before it is spoken, but he can only get to his target by repeated trial-and-error attempts. He may be very good at quickly self-correcting his spoken mistakes, but he makes them repeatedly.

Some aphasics have a "yes-no" confusion; they frequently will say "yes" when they mean "no," and vice versa, even nodding or shaking their heads for the unwanted response. Unless people are alerted to this, the patient may have what seems to be unreasonable emotional flare-ups after he has been given something he had apparently agreed he wanted.

There is an occasional patient who is not heard to utter a sound during the early weeks following onset of aphasia. This patient is either very dysarthric or may have an extremely severe form of apraxia of speech. He is often in great fear, prohibiting attempts at sound production, and his understanding of speech may be so poor that no one can explain to him what is happening or what he should try to do. It is very important for a voiceless patient to be examined by a speech pathologist as early as possible, as there are ways to stimulate voice for many of them.

What Can Be Done About Aphasics Who Use Profanity Liberally? Why Do They Do It?

When a sweet, aphasic, elderly lady, who has never been known to utter four-letter words or profanities in her entire life, has one or more such expressions fall from her lips whenever she tries to say something, the listener's reaction is often, to say the least, one of surprise. It can be a startling experience, even embarrassing to some family members, to hear these words produced repeatedly by someone who cannot seem to say anything else that has meaning. Nurses and other paramedical personnel working with these patients may become offended and make every effort to put a stop to the utterances.

As stated earlier, this is a form of automatic speech. For certain neurological and, perhaps, emotional reasons, there seems to be a direct route to these words stored somewhere in the brain of certain patients, and most efforts to talk will activate production of these particular words whereas all other words cannot be elicited. Interestingly enough, they are used no more often by aphasics than "dee dee dee" or other automatic and repetitive productions, but because of the strong impact on the ears of some listeners, they seem to be more common, whereas they may actually be less so.

Listeners do not try to stop patients from other benign but repetitive automatic expressions, but the profane or the four-letter words are often greeted with horror, anger, and even threats. I have seen many a battle waged by non-speech pathology professionals, by family members, or by friends, trying in vain to put an end to what they consider to be intolerable obscenities.

To try to shut them off before a patient has regained some ability to produce meaningful words at will is unwise and unfair. By far the kindest as well as the most sensible course to follow is to ignore them; in fact, since it is possible to strengthen the tendency just by calling attention to it, there is a better chance of reducing the occurrences if no attention is paid to them. If, however, ignoring the words proves unbearable to some listeners, it would probably be in the patient's best interest if these people turned their duties over to others with more tolerance for this behavior.

Can It Help to Ask an Aphasic the Names of Things Around Him?

When an aphasic reaches the level where he can name things correctly about 80 percent of the time without imitating someone saying the word or without some kind of cue, then it is very helpful to have him do this regularly. Before he reaches that level, however, it is not only useless, but can be of emotional harm to him because of the frustration and feelings of failure it is bound to induce. In the next section some guidelines will be presented for helping him regain the process of naming objects, if he has the potential to do so.

How Can He Be Helped to Find the Word He Wants to Say?

The first step is to name objects to him *without expecting him to say anything*. This is a step that may need to be followed for days, weeks, or even months before another step can be added. One purpose for this is to reactivate the names of things that he has not been able to retrieve. Those patients who have no difficulty at this level should not be held back to it, but most aphasic patients will have some word-finding problems, especially in the early days after onset. It is an easy enough task to accomplish. Anyone in contact with him for even a few minutes, long enough perhaps to bring him a breakfast tray, can be very helpful by merely saying: "Breakfast." And by pointing a moment to each item as it is named: "Cereal, toast, coffee, milk." Single words are more meaningful at this stage than long, involved cheery speeches. The nurse who comes in with an energetic: "Good morning. It's time to eat now. Let's see what we have for you today," is providing a fine greeting for people who understand well and can talk, but to the aphasic these words may sound a bit different from the way they were meant. He may hear something like: "Goo ahm. Ty eeow. See shee ot foo ay." Not only is this meaningless jargon to this particular aphasic, but it is utterly useless for him in any therapeutic sense. In that same brief space of time, the nurse could be providing him with a start toward recovering some language ability "Hi . . . breakfast . . . eat . . . eggs . . . juice," etc. as she points to each item. As each separate word, with its object indicated, is transmitted to the brain, there is a good chance that it will reinforce the word stored there with its meaning, and sooner or later the aphasic may be able to retrieve it at will. This simple technique is very effective in stimulating memory of words and their meanings for many aphasic patients.

Naming should not be limited to food, of course. The names of people close to him, even those of his wife and children, may have to be offered repeatedly before he recalls them himself. It is to many aphasics a shameful secret that they do not recall the names of their loved ones; for some even the word "wife" is lost. Body parts should be named; while they are being washed and thus stimulated tactually is a particularly fine time to name them. The date and day should be spoken to him daily, not only to stimulate the words, but to try to keep him in touch with the passage of time if any of the words can penetrate with meaning. Many aphasics are shocked—when they do become aware of time much later—that months have passed that they did not note. In many hospital wards now the date and day are clearly printed in large letters daily, because it is so easy for hospitalized patients to lose track of time, and the aphasic patient who cannot read the paper is even more likely than others to be totally unaware of its passage.

The next step may be added as soon as the patient is able to do it. This step is one in which he is asked to imitate a word spoken to him. The word should be one that has been used in the naming exercise. If his understanding is fairly good, he may respond correctly just by being asked to repeat what is said to him. Many patients, however, will require repetitions of the instructions, perhaps a rephrasing of them. Gestures may be needed to get the point across, in the following way: first point to an object directly before the patient, let us say a cup. Say the word "cup" while pointing to one's mouth. Then point to the patient's mouth repeating: "Say 'cup.'" If he says it successfully, he must be told that it was right, with a show of approval, because many aphasics cannot tell if they have said something correctly and need this kind of feedback in order to retrieve their own self-critical ability. Care must be taken not to overdo the praise, as that can be a source of disturbance to him. Just enough praise to guide him in the direction of success is what is needed, but not so much as to appear gushy and inappropriate.

Aphasics with no other complications generally have no trouble repeating the words spoken to them, once they understand what is wanted of them. Those who have apraxia and/or dysarthria may not be able to imitate well, or at all. In that case, the chapters on these conditions must be studied carefully before attempting to go further with retrieval of speaking ability (Chapters X and XI). Repeating the word correctly and endowing it with its meaning are two quite different skills. Therefore, it is very important to connect the spoken word with its object or a picture of it whenever this exercise is used.

During this period, the same words should be used with the exercises presented in Chapter IV, in which understanding of the word was the drill. A period of time may be divided among the different tasks in this way: (1) a word is spoken to him and the speaker points to the object or picture; (2) when three or four of these are done, the patient is asked to point to the one named; (3) the word is spoken again and he is asked to imitate it while he or the speaker points to the object. When these combined tasks are correctly performed most of the time, as many as ten objects can be presented for one session.

It is good to keep a diary of the number of successes and failures he has during each dated session. When he is successfully able to imitate correctly and point to the right object at least 90 percent, or better, 100 percent of the time, another step can be added. Keeping such a diary of scores also documents growth. Sometimes improvement is so slow that only by reviewing these dated records does the positive proof of growth emerge, and this can be rewarding when discouragement sets in as it often does for both the patient and those close to him.

When he is ready for the next step, one good technique is to use open-ended sentences which the speaker supplies and for which the patient is required to provide the final word—one of the words used in the previous exercises. Such a sentence must be carefully framed so only the desired word is the one likely to be chosen. For example, "My wife's name is ————" is obviously a good choice. "I drink coffee out of a ————," "To eat soup from a bowl, we use a ————," etc. It is good to have the pictures or objects in sight so they can also be used as a stimulus in addition to the sentence spoken until he can do this task well. It is even a good idea to provide the required word for the patient to imitate the first few times this exercise is presented, but if he cannot say the word alone, without a model, after the sentence is presented open-endedly several more times, he is probably not ready for this step.

The open-ended sentence is but one form of cue that may be used to elicit the desired word. Long known and well-learned proverbs can be useful, such as "A bird in the hand is worth two in the ————," "Be it ever so humble, there's no place like ————." There are distinct advantages to using statements that were well learned many years earlier, as these are not so apt to be affected by the brain injury as more recently learned material. Lines from nursery rhymes would be particularly good except that some patients are insulted and threatened by such juvenile material. Those who can handle this type of material without emotional reaction find that the ease of recall it provides makes it especially valuable.

When he is successful 90 percent or 100 percent of the time with cues alone, without a model, a new step may be added. None of the preceding steps should be dropped when a new one is added; rather, new material should be introduced to the earlier steps.

The final step of this task is the actual naming of the object by the patient without a model and without a cue other than the object or picture itself. He is asked to say what each is called as the person working with him points to the object, perhaps saying to him, "This is a ————." Thus only by painstakingly going through these steps does the proper time arrive when it is profitable and safe to ask an aphasic to name objects and people around him.

Verbs need to be handled in similar fashion but it is necessary to provide pictures of people clearly performing certain actions in order to elicit the words like walk, jump, run, sleep, and so on. Imitation, pointing to the picture of the action after the words are spoken, and providing the word in an open-ended sentence such as "The man (walks)," "The girl (eats)" are the steps before he is asked to provide the verb alone without a model or cue to describe action in a picture. It is necessary to keep in mind that communication, not intact grammar, is the immediate goal; therefore the correct tense is not an issue here, but rather the correct verb in any of its forms.

After retrieving some nouns and verbs, working with prepositions is important. To be able to say the name of the object one has in mind and to provide the word standing for the action performed by or to that object are big steps toward restoring communicative ability, but a further step can be taken when a word describing position of the object can be added, such as on, under, in, around, and behind. Adjectives, especially those of position such as right and left, are good to introduce. In all of these words, the meaning must precede the spoken word, because it is of no value for the aphasic to utter a group of sounds that are meaningless to him even though they add up to a real word to the listener.

For some people it is helpful to provide printed words, about a half inch in height, along with the picture or object. These are additional cues that may elicit and reinforce what is sought. For others it is of no value to provide this and may even be a deterring factor if he tries too hard to make sense out of the written form and is thus distracted from the basic task. Those patients who read and understand the written word easily are best helped by the addition of this material.

Introduction of phrases and sentences to be spoken by the aphasic needs to be very carefully handled. A short sentence such as "I am happy" or "I am mad" is immediately useful and so can be self-reinforcing. "I want ————" followed by likely interests of each person should be taken into consideration when choices of words for drill are made. Words that are of immediate practical and emotional appeal will be used more frequently and therefore become habitual sooner than words that the patient is not likely to need daily.

It is certainly not intended that each word the patient is ever going to be able to say again must be painstakingly drilled this way. If this were true speech therapy would be too burdensome ever to undertake. The goal with these tasks, as with all attempts to improve communication, is to retrieve functions and processes that were blocked by the injury. Not all will be restored, but only by trying to revive them will it be possible to determine what can be regained. As each task is drilled and some words become habitual, certain clusters of words may begin to emerge without any drill, complete with meaning. These are exciting occurrences, for the patient and for his listeners.

Should Faulty Pronunciation and Other Errors Be Corrected?

When speech is just being introduced and retrieved, getting the patient's idea across to the listener is the most important aspect of talking. It matters little whether he uses plurals for singulars, present tense for past, or even if he includes all the syllables in a multisyllabic word whose meaning is clear, such as "hamburg" for "hamburger" when he orders his lunch. Early use of words should stress only meaning; that involves providing the word that means what he wants to say so others get his message. Much later, if he becomes fluent in ability to express himself but persists in mispronunciations, in grammatical and syntactical errors, etc., that is the time to be concerned with these issues and to use drill sessions to work on them. Requiring perfection too soon may cut off incentive to speak enough for improvement to take place.

Is It Wise to Pretend to Understand Him When He Is Not Understood?

It can prevent improvement if people pretend they understand a patient's jargon and incorrect, automatic speech. An aphasic who thinks he is well understood has no incentive to try to learn to speak meaningfully. He may become furious when people do not respond correctly to his requests, not realizing they are not comprehended but thinking, instead, that his wishes are being ignored. A patient I knew who had originally used only jargon but thought he was speaking correctly, later described to me the early days following his brain hemorrhage. He would lie in bed in the hospital asking his wife and others to get him a bedpan. They would smile and nod, and perhaps pat his arm, and chat away at him or with one another, making no effort to comply with his requests. He had no inkling that they did not understand him. They listened when he spoke, and their facial expressions seemed receptive enough, but no response was forthcoming. At first he was very angry; later he became confused and then frightened. He could not understand the behavior of all these familiar people who spoke strange sounds at and around him, laughed and smiled, yet made no move to carry out his simplest wish. A speech pathologist was finally consulted and was the first one to make it known to him by gestures, shrugs, hands outspread regretfully, shaking of the head, that his words were not getting across. The original impact of this discovery was of more fear, but when he realized the therapist was going to help him learn to talk correctly, the relief was intense, and the incentive to cooperate was strong.

His wife described to me her view of those early days. She was afraid to let him know she did not understand him, so she nodded eagerly at all he said. She had no realization that he was not understanding her and so she chattered away telling him all the news of home and family, trying to keep it light and pleasant by laughing at some of the anecdotes she told. When he would suddenly appear to be very angry, even throwing things on the floor or lashing out at her and others, her concern was great. He was labeled as uncooperative by the staff, and there was even some talk of perhaps having to put him into a locked facility eventually. He was put on a tranquilizing medication that interferred with his ability to concentrate in speech therapy, but later, when the medication was discontinued, he was able to profit from treatment. His wife was at first disturbed when the therapist let him know that his speech was unintelligible. This seemed to her unnecessary cruelty, until the reasons for this action were made clear and she saw the effects knowing the truth had upon his behavior.

Some people feel they must listen to the patient indefinitely while he is trying unsuccessfully, with many false starts and stops, to get a point across. Family members, particularly when they first bring a patient home from the hospital, are apt to spend a great deal of time trying to make sense out of what the patient is saying, usually with poor results. The effect upon both is often extreme fatigue, frustration, and hopelessness. When the meaning does not come through after a short period of trying, it is best to indicate to him through gestures, as well as words, that although it is very regretable, he is not understandable at this time. If he cannot get his point across by gestures, pictures, drawings, or use of a communication notebook (to be described later), the only sensible thing to do is to give it up at that time, before everyone is worn out. There are some patients who learn that they can keep the center of attention by trying to talk, so they will make these futile attempts whenever they can find people willing to stay with them indefinitely. Soon people learn to avoid them as much as possible, and the end result is very self-defeating.

There is no doubt that, sometimes, by staying with a patient while he tries, by trial and error, to make himself understood, some very important need is finally expressed. Recently a patient who generally gave up when his attempts were not productive, stubbornly refused to be thwarted on one particular occasion; so I stayed with him until, after nearly ten minutes of fumbles, reversals, perseverations, and all the rest, he was able to let me know that he needed an attorney for a very urgent personal matter. After enough time is spent with a patient, his behavior patterns can be more or less recognized, so that when it is important for him to get a message out, others can be alerted that this time they had better try to understand, and spend more time trying.

Is Singing of Any Value to Aphasics?

Some aphasics can perfectly sing the words to music of songs they have known almost all their lives. Then, when some of those same words are needed in speech a short time later, they cannot produce them. The probable reason for this phenomenon is that the words to the songs were stored, along with the music, in a different part of the brain—the right hemisphere—and were not damaged or cut off from retrieval when the left hemisphere language centers were injured. It is a very puzzling, mystifying experience to hear an aphasic sing a song, sometimes very clearly and correctly, and not be able to say the same phrases or sentences without the music. Not all aphasics can do this, and the reasons are not clear why some can and some cannot.

Whether or not it helps him to recover language if he is encouraged to sing is also not entirely known. There is a form of treatment in which the aphasic is encouraged to chant the words he tries to say to a sort of tune. Some speech pathologists have reported a certain amount of success with this method used with some patients.

It is good to have as many techniques available to stimulate language recovery as possible. What works with one patient may not work with another. Therefore, if a patient does not refuse to sing, encouraging singing is a fine thing to do, if only for the relaxing pleasure it can bring. Some patients can only hum along or provide a partial attempt at a word here and there, and among these, with enough attempts, words sometimes emerge later. Some patients love singing the old, long known songs like "Row, Row, Row Your Boat," and among these, a few are able to carry the words over into speech to a certain extent. Newer, more recently learned songs do not seem to work as well, but they are worth trying.

What Should Be Done When He Keeps Repeating the Same Word Although Trying to Say Something Else?

Perseveration, or repetition of a word that is not appropriate even if it was first used correctly, is a common form of automatic speech. Some patients perseverate on the same word for days, weeks, months, and even years. Others come up with a repeated word during one period of a day and emerge with another one later. Here it helps to know the speech behavior of the patient in order to handle this well. For the type of patient described earlier who self-monitors his speech effectively and can self-correct his errors, it is appropriate to give him plenty of time to work his way through all the perseverations and detours until he gets to his goal. If what he is trying to say becomes evident to the listener, it can spare both patient and audience much time and discomfort by asking if that is what he wants to say and providing him with a model. Sometimes giving the correct word is enough to break through the perseveration. At other times the new word becomes a new perseveration.

If the patient is known to have little success trying to break through perseverations and emerge with any meaning, it is wise to try to divert his attention. There is some evidence that the more often an incorrect response is repeated the more likely it is to get fixed and resistant to a correct one. It might be good to tell him lightly, with regrets, that perhaps he had better listen for a while or watch television or take a walk and try again later. Telling him a diverting story that requires no verbal response from him is a good tactic if he understands well enough. The patient who goes on in this type of a perseverative circle needs help to turn off the behavior: "Get me some light, no-uh, light--no, no-uh, I mean, yes that's it, -uh, light, no -uh-light, no, no, no." This can go on indefinitely with never a clue to what he is trying to say. The kindest thing to do is to get him into a different form of behavior from speech: listening, walking, eating, etc., but this must not be done as an order or punishment. It is important that the patient does not get the feeling that he is being shut up because he has failed or has become a nuisance. If possible, he should be made to feel that by leaving the words for a while, they have a good chance to correct themselves later, and that the listener very much wants to hear what he has to say.

What Should Be Done When an Aphasic Cannot Say Something He Said Well Earlier?

This is a frequent question. If the listener thinks he understands what the patient is trying to say, he might ask him if that is the word he is seeking. If so, it is good to provide him with the word as a model for imitation several times. For patients with good understanding, discussing the frustrations of aphasia, calling it by name and describing how apparent it is that he can say the word sometimes and not others, can be a very rewarding discussion. Empathizing with his frustration at not being able to depend on his word recall ability can help him feel less isolated.

How Can Others Help Him to Communicate More Easily?

This section contains some repetitions from other sections, but it is appropriate to present them again here as basic principles.

1. Give him plenty of time to say what he is trying to say when it is clear that by giving him time he has a good chance at success. Many aphasics need time to process in order to find the word; some require stumbling, repetitions, self-corrections, or even cues from the listener who thinks he knows what is coming. When the patient habitually has few successes, do not allow him to get into the habit of remaining "on stage" with repeated failures.

2. It is all right for the listener to guess what he is trying to say, but it is not all right for the listener to speak for him all the time. Too many family members get into a habit of speaking for the patient whenever other people are around; perhaps the intent is loving but the results are negative. "John loves to watch the game on TV, don't you John? He is very fond of steak and we'll have that for dinner tonight, won't we, John? He is so happy to see you. He'd like you to visit again soon, don't you, John?" Patients in this situation usually make no attempt to talk when others are around except for their immediate family. Perhaps they sense that the main reason for all the talk is to cover up embarrassment that others are feeling, an embarrassment that might become more intense if he were to try and fail to say something properly.

3. Do not insist that words or grammar be correctly spoken. Communication, not perfection, is the goal. Social times should not be therapy time. If certain words appear to be stumbling blocks, they can be noted and worked on at the next session of home or professional treatment, but never when conversation is social during periods of relaxation.

4. Praise for his efforts and for every sign of new success is important, but must not be overdone. Some aphasics become depressed by too much praise for \what they see as going back to early childhood when they were first learning to talk. Praise should always be honestly given. Improvement needs praise as much as successful production; this can help shape the desired behavior and point it in the right direction. He should be told—if he understands—when he does something that he was unable to do previously. When a behavior becomes habitual it must no longer be praised. I cringe with patients who must endure gushingly produced approbation, unable as they are to say "Knock it off!" A simple "Good! You said that well" is usually enough recognition.

5. Promises of his future ability to talk perfectly again must *never* be made to him. Except to say that he will get better, it is best to keep the focus on actual improvement up to the present rather than some future fantasized goal that no one can deliver. Some family members feel that if they do not

promise that all will be fine again one day, the patient will give up entirely. That is not so. There is a difference between taking away all hope and promising the moon. No patient should ever be told that he will never improve, that this is the way he will talk forever, but neither should he be told that he will be as good as new. Continued improvement is as far as anyone can go in making predictions.

6. Never pretend to understand him when his speech is not intelligible.

7. Some family members think that the patient needs to be protected against social contact with others and should be treated as an invalid for the rest of his life. I have actually found aphasic patients, years after onset, who are kept to their rooms when visitors come. There is no doubt that a warm, loving, humorous family, in which the aphasic is completely accepted, to which friends return again and again as they always did, where patience, honest relationships, and fun are greatly evident, provides the most desirable setting for an aphasic to recover language to the utmost of his potential. Most of us fall short of being able to provide this ideal setting. Yet keeping in mind a picture of what is most desirable, an attempt can be made to approach it. The patient *needs* social contact. Keeping him in isolation, with only his physical needs tended, will cause him to regress or fall short of his potential.

8. No one should be demanding or critical of his attempts to communicate. He should not be forced to talk, but should be given ample opportunity to do so when with others.

9. If he can use gestures well enough to enhance his word-meaning he should be encouraged or even *taught* to do so (see Chapter VIII).

10. If he can draw pictures of what he is trying to say, he should be encouraged to use this means.

11. If he can write, even a little, a few letters may convey the meaning of what he is trying to say with partially articulated words. For example, if he is trying to say that he is thirsty but the words do not form in any way that their meaning can be interpreted, by writing "wat" on paper he may convey that he wants a drink of water. Patients who are mainly apraxic and only very mildly aphasic can often write much better than they can talk, and should always have with them something to write on.

12. A communication notebook or chart should be provided when he has great trouble producing intelligible speech (discussed below).

What Is a Communication Notebook and How Can It Help?

The purpose of a communication notebook is to enable a person who has limited ability to speak or write to convey messages to others. Each notebook must be made up to suit the individual needs of one patient, so they cannot be bought ready made.

A large loose-leaf notebook is a good place to start, and a few good, colored pictures of the most urgent situations or the most important people he might want to indicate can be pasted on the first pages. The name of each should be printed or written in large letters beneath each picture. Pictures of a toilet, glass of water, cup of coffee, or any other special food or drink he likes and might be wanting should be added. Pictures of family members are especially important when he is in a hospital away from his loved ones, and he cannot say their names to his nurses or therapists. In this case ages and birthdays might be added to the names of children and grandchildren, plus some personal item about each, so others can mention these to the patient.

If he has any special hobby or interests, pictures of these should be used. A fisherman should have pictures of fish, types of tackle, boats, and so on. Learning to say the names of items that have special emotional impact for him is a great motivation in recovering speech. This is one reason that flash cards used randomly are not as valuable as screening the cards to select appropriate pictures, or collecting magazine pictures of special items important to the patient. However, it takes many magazines to produce the variety of pictures needed for one patient. It is not only expensive to collect magazines, but it is very time consuming to find suitable pictures. Enlisting the help of others who volunteer their services is worthwhile. If enough pictures cannot be collected this way, flashcards can be bought at bookstores that sell material for helping children learn to read, or a speech pathologist can suggest where they can be purchased.

Some aphasics are not able to make use of a communication notebook. They cannot learn to find the correct picture or even to point dependably to what they want to talk about. Until it is determined with a few pictures that the patient can use them adequately, an elaborate notebook should not be created. Some may need training to learn to use it to convey meaning. If a patient enjoys a cup of coffee, for example, a picture of a steaming cup of this liquid may be used. Then the person training him can take his hand and point with it to the picture saying, "Oh, you want a cup of coffee," and he should get a real one immediately. Any attempt of his to use the notebook should be rewarded with immediate attention and correct responses.

Chapter VI

Aphasia: Reading

Do All Aphasics Have Reading Problems?
If He Reads Aloud Perfectly Does That Prove He
Understands What He Reads?
If He Appears to Enjoy Reading Newspapers and Letters
Does That Prove He Has No Reading Problem?
Can a Reading Problem Be Helped with Glasses or a
Change of Prescription?
What Visual Difficulties Other than Aphasia Can Be
Caused by Brain Injury?
How Can His Reading Ability and Other Visual Status Be
Determined?
What Are Some Ways to Help Him Improve His Reading
Ability?

Do All Aphasics Have Reading Problems?

A few very fortunate people have no change in their reading ability with onset of aphasia. These are generally apt to be those whose aphasia is so mild from the start that they will return to completely normal language ability in a few months. Most others have reading problems. There is as wide a variety in the type of reading problems found in aphasia as in the other language areas; difficulties range from very mild, moderate, severe, to total inability to read anything at all.

Some people have a memory disorder which produces what appears to be a reading disability. These people cannot remember much of what they read so that by the time they have read through a short paragraph they have forgotten how it started. They cannot be interested in reading a book or even a newspaper article because they cannot retain enough to develop any continuity. The husband of a patient of mine kept bringing her books to read, which she rejected. She had always been an avid reader and there was no doubt that she read and understood words and sentences in the books; therefore, her husband could not understand her refusal to read newspapers, magazies, and books. Testing of her memory for recent input revealed that it was seriously impaired and at that time reading could be of no value to her. With a great deal of work on memory she improved in the following months and could read short stories and articles with interest. Not everyone can improve.

Some aphasics understand nouns or verbs but do not understand any of the "little" words, the pronouns, prepositions, conjunctions, and articles. If all these words are obliterated from a page a normal reader tries to read, it soon becomes apparent that without them the meaning of the material is very unclear. The reader might have an idea of what the subject of the material is, but has no idea what really happened to it. If all the nouns or verbs are erased, the problem becomes even more acute.

Many aphasics substitute words as they read and thereby lose or change the meaning entirely. Others omit words they actually know, or they add words, again causing the meaning to be altered.

There are many aphasics who cannot read at all. The letters themselves have lost all meaning. Some people lose this ability when the remaining language areas are only mildly or moderately impaired. A very severely impaired aphasic will have no more ability to make any sense out of the written word than he has in understanding the speech of others, or in trying to speak or write.

If He Reads Aloud Perfectly Does That Prove He Understands What He Reads?

There are some aphasics who read aloud perfectly, even with inflection at times, and who do not understand a single word they have read. These same words can be spoken to them by others and they may understand them well when they hear others say them, depending upon their ability to comprehend speech, but meaning seems to have become disconnected from the words when read aloud or silently by themselves. To test this, a card may be given to this aphasic, with instructions which may read: "Pick up the book" or "Touch your nose." It is a fascinating and mystifying phenomenon when this person reads the words aloud correctly over and over, shaking his head and finally giving up, unable to derive any meaning from the words he has read aloud with perfect ability.

There are a few aphasics who can write but cannot read. Therefore they can write a letter or some other material but have no ability to read back what they have written. Reading, as in each of the other language skills, is not one smooth function but rather a combination of functions that are so well coordinated in normal readers that they seem to act as one. Any part or parts that break down may leave all the others intact. This is how it can come about that some aphasics can read aloud very well with no comprehension at all of what they read.

If He Appears to Enjoy Reading Newspapers or Letters Does That Prove He Has No Reading Problem?

There are patients who insist on reading the daily paper and seem to read eagerly all the cards and letters they receive, yet testing of their reading ability reveals that they understand perhaps 20 percent of the simple nouns and 10 percent of verbs and few other parts of speech. When I tell their families that their reading is very impaired, they disagree strongly and describe how much the patient enjoys reading. I will then demonstrate by means of various testing techniques how little the patient actually understands of what he seems to do so well.

Some aphasics insist on "reading" everything in sight even when only a few words here and there emerge meaningfully. They seem to want to keep trying, perhaps finding that over time more and more words being to make sense. Moreover, they may actually obtain enough of an idea of what is written that they feel they really understand it. They may correctly read the signature on a card or letter and thus feel closer to that person if they glean some information from the words he has written, even if most of the letter remains meaningless.

I know a little French and when I am in that country I enjoy trying to understand something in their newspapers or magazines, yet I must confess that most of the material remains untranslatable to me. Anyone watching me pore over the pages would certainly believe that I knew how to read French well. So with these aphasic patients who appear to read well when they have a notable reading disability.

It is necessary for others to understand the real reading limitations of an aphasic patient. If it is assumed that he has no problem, no one will seek ways to try to help him improve. Furthermore, an important decision may need his concurrence. If he is given a key document to read and the family believes his response to be based on good understanding of that document, an erroneous conclusion may be reached. This actually occurred to a family I knew. They finally sought help when they had a near disaster based on their complete misunderstanding of their father's ability to understand documents given to him for approval, as well as their strong overestimation of his ability to understand what they said to him.

Can a Reading Problem Be Helped with Glasses or a Change of Prescription?

Aphasic reading problems cannot be helped by glasses. Aphasic patients who can benefit from getting glasses, either for the first time or for a different correction, are those who needed these changes before the brain injury and had not provided for them. If there was any suspicion before the onset of aphasia that he was due for different glasses, this needs to be brought to the attention of his physician and speech pathologist.

Reading test results cannot be accurate if the glasses are incorect or missing when the patient is tested. Since testing of aphasia must include a reading test to be complete, it is important to have the proper glasses at the time of the test. Inability to understand what is being read, inability to know the meaning of letters or words, is caused by the brain injury, not by distorted vision. The printed words can be blown up to large size so there is no doubt that the aphasic can see them clearly, yet if he is unable to comprehend the meaning, the words will remain meaningless.

What Visual Difficulties Other than Aphasia Can Be Caused by Brain Injury?

Some patients lose part of the vision in each eye. These are called *visual field cuts* and are actually areas of blindness. Thus a patient with paralysis on the right side of his body may also lose visual fields in the right side of both eyes. This does not mean that he is blind in his right eye, but rather that he has blind areas on the right side of both left and right eyes. Many of these patients are unaware of this new inability to see things on their far right, so they do not compensate for this by turning their head further to the right. They will be apt to miss seeing objects on that side; they may knock over unseen glasses of water, bump into doorways or walls, and, if they drive, may have serious accidents. In addition to blindness to things on their right, they also have a blind area that would include those things normally seen by the right side of their left eye. This leads to varying kinds of difficulties with vision. Even if they can read fairly well, they may miss entire sections of words on the right side of the page and therefore misunderstand what they are reading.

New glasses can be of no help to patients with this kind of deficit. These patients are often seen rubbing their eyes or wiping their glasses thinking something is on the lens, or they may discard them altogether thinking they are causing the problem.

A patient with a visual field cut needs to be trained to compensate for his new difficulty. If he understands well enough, his visual problem can be explained to him and he must learn to turn his head further to the right than he is accustomed to turning it. We have all become conditioned to turning our heads a certain amount to make up for the normal limits of our peripheral vision. The aphasic with a right visual field cut needs to be carefully retrained to turn his head regularly further to the right. Unfortunately many of these patients have poor memories and therefore cannot easily learn to make this adjustment, so walls get gouged by wheelchairs and many table cloths get soaked before the learning takes effect. As for those who can read, many people have found that if a vertical bright red line is drawn down the right side of a page of printed material, they are more easily trained to continue reading until that line is reached.

Another type of problem many aphasic patients encounter is a visual-spatial difficulty. They cannot keep their eyes fixed on the line they are reading; therefore, they insert words from above or below, obviously completely changing the meaning of the material. Some will skip lines and omit entire sections of a paragraph. Even if their comprehension for reading words is undamaged, they will receive faulty information by skipping or inserting words, so they are not likely to read with good understanding of the material. Glasses cannot help this kind of problem. What can help some patients is a card held under each line so they follow along in the proper sequence, or better still a card with a window cut out the size of one line of print, so their eyes cannot skip to lines above the one they are reading. However, patients with a tremor in their good hand may have difficulty controlling the card when they try to move it down from line to line.

There are some patients who develop double vision as a result of brain injury. All visual tasks become extremely difficult, and reading or writing are often impossible. An eye doctor or a neurologist with special knowledge of visual problems should be consulted so that the proper measures are taken to deal with this problem.

How Can His Reading Ability and Other Visual Status Be Determined?

A physician can determine if he has visual field cuts, inability to keep his eyes in focus, or double vision. A speech pathologist experienced in treating adult aphasia is the most efficient professional for testing his reading ability.

If a speech pathologist is not available to the patient, a superficial screening of his ability to understand words can be undertaken in a home treatment program. For this, ten nouns can be printed or written in large letters, each on a separate card. The objects represented by the nouns should be placed on a table before the patient and the cards placed beside each object it names. Simple, familiar items must be used, such as a cup, a watch, a book, a glass, and so on. When he has had a chance to look at the cards and objects carefully, all but two or three should be removed and the cards for those items carefully mixed. One at a time a card should be handed to him after telling him to put the card by the correct object, using gestures along with words if there is reason to suspect that he may not understand the spoken words. If he places these cards correctly add more objects until all ten are used at that session.

The purpose of this test is to learn if the aphasic understands these simple nouns all the time, some of the time, or not at all. He may know 20 percent or 50 percent or 75 percent of them. He may fluctuate so that at one time he knows 30 percent and the next only 10 percent. He may need processing time, that is, time to read the card over and over until the meaning emerges. Some will place a card on an incorrect object, then later realize the error and correct it. Some will merely shake their heads in sad bewilderment, indicating that the words are meaningless. Others may just place all the cards in a pile or put them on the wrong objects without realizing their error. There are many patterns and each must be dealt with differently.

If he has no trouble with the nouns, a more difficult task needs to be tried next. Using the same object, a card may read, "Put this card on the one used for drinking," "Put this card under the one used for reading," or "Put this card to the left of the book." There are many ways to test various parts of speech, and if done properly, a clear picture of the aphasic's reading ability will emerge.

It is good to document his reading test results so that when the test is given again a month or two later, progress can be duly noted. The general trend during the early months is toward progress, in reading as in all other language skills. An aphasic who understood 25 percent of the nouns and no prepositions at one month after onset may, three months later, understand 50 percent of them and, perhaps, 20 percent of the prepositions. Without documentation it is easy to overlook evidence of progress.

When an aphasic has no difficulty with individual words or the brief sentences on the cards, longer sentences should be used in a variety of situations, using words that he understands in the simpler sentences. The purpose now is to learn whether he can retain meaning when it becomes more complex. For example, two of the earlier tasks can be combined on one card so he will read, "Put the book under the cup and the spoon in the cup," or "Touch your nose with your finger after you pick up the watch."

If these tasks are successfully carried out, then a very short story may be presented to him for his silent reading. A list of written questions pertaining to the story is then given to him. They must be worded in such a way that he only has to check if they are right or wrong. If he misses many of the points of the story it can be concluded that he cannot retain enough information to read a newspaper or book with good comprehension.

It is best to have him perform all the reading test tasks with silent reading only. Those patients who have any speech problem, no matter how minor, should not use speech when their reading ability is being tested, neither to read the material nor to provide the answers to questions. It is important in all testing of aphasic patients to avoid as much as possible using a defective language skill to test another defective skill. That is not always possible, as so much information must be given to the patient through speech, and if he has poor understanding of speech, his failure to do the task may be due to his inability to understand what was expected of him rather than actual inability to perform.

What Are Some Ways to Help Him Improve His Reading Ability?

Before any attempt is made to help him with reading, the exact nature of his reading disability must be determined. In addition, there are certain other important things to consider, such as *when* to work on it.

In treatment of aphasia, certain language skills take precedence over others in helping the patient improve. Work attempted too soon in one area may be wasted time, or more seriously, harmful because of the frustration resulting from attempting an activity prematurely. Understanding the speech of others, with few exceptions, generally takes precedence with most patients over all other language disabilities. In many cases, just working on and improving the speech comprehension problems produces an improvement in reading without any direct work done with reading itself.

If a patient is severely or moderately aphasic so that he understands little of what is said to him and has great difficulty making himself understood with his speech, he is in no way ready to begin work on reading. If, however, his comprehension of what is said to him is good or only mildly impaired, he may be ready to benefit from reading therapy even if he has difficulty talking (which may be due to apraxia of speech rather than aphasia).

It is necessary to know if there are any visual problems in addition to aphasia that may interfere with reading. Furthermore, if a patient refuses to work on reading, his wishes must be respected. Only he can know subjectively what discomforts he experiences when attempting to read.

Before starting a program he must be carefully tested to determine just where to start. As in all language therapy, treatment should start just where the patient is beginning to have problems. If the testing revealed that he understands some nouns, that is the place to start, not with sentences or more abstract parts of speech. If, however, he understands no nouns but does know some verbs, it is best to start with verbs. The same kinds of cards may be used that were used in the test, carefully avoiding test objects, however, because when the test is repeated at a later date, the same cards should be used as in the original test. If the test items are used in therapy they may actually be learned, although temporarily, and a true picture of reading improvement cannot be obtained. Either objects or pictures of objects can be used with their names on the cards. If action pictures are used when verbs are selected as the task, the verb is printed on the card instead of the noun. When working on prepositions, the card can read simply: "on the chair" or "under the box." The patient's desired response is to place the cards according to what the words mean, for example, "Run," by a picture of a boy running.

Until a patient reaches 90 percent or 100 percent competency in a particular step, he must not be introduced to a harder level of reading material. Many patients will never be able to progress beyond the one-word level in reading; therefore, by becoming impatient and introducing a more difficult task before he is competent in the earlier one, his ultimate potential for reading recovery may be passed. It is better to continue to work below a patient's optimal level than to exceed it and try to push him into areas he cannot possibly handle.

When a patient becomes competent in enough parts of speech and sentences so that he can be introduced to paragraphs, his memory span must be carefully checked. If that seems to present no problem and he handles paragraphs well, which is learned by his checking correctly true and false questions presented after every paragraph, then he may be ready for short stories or newspaper articles. At any point where the testing reveals that he is not understanding well, it is best to back-track and build up again to the level where he began to break down. Daily fluctuations require no progression beyond that point until or unless stabilization of responses occurs.

Patients who reach a level where they can read articles and books but still feel a lack of former competency, must keep reading a great deal to improve their skills. Sometimes they can be helped in adult education classes or by using textbooks of 4th grade reading level and above to strengthen certain basic skills whose weakness may be interfering with their progress. Not many aphasics will regain their former ability, but those who reach the levels where reading for pleasure is once again possible have every reason to keep trying to improve their skills.

Chapter VII

Aphasia: Writing

Do All Aphasics Have Writing Problems?
Is Writing Difficult Because He Has To Use His
Unaccustomed Hand?
If He Cannot Use Speech Effectively Is Writing a Good
Substitute?
If He Cannot Write, Is a Typewriter a Good Substitute?
Can Spelling Boards and Spelling Games Such as Scrabble
and Crossword Puzzles Be of Help?
Can He Recover Ability to Spell and to Use Grammar and
Syntax Correctly in Writing?
How Can He Be Helped to Improve His Writing
Ability?

Do All Aphasics Have Writing Problems?

With few exceptions, all aphasics have writing problems, especially in the early period following onset. The person with only a mild aphasia at the start may complain that he cannot recall a word he is trying to write, just as he finds some words elusive when he tries to say them. He may become irritated that the spelling of simple words seems to come out wrong at times, but with concentrated effort he can usually solve the problem. In a few months this person often finds that he has no more difficulty with writing than he does with other language areas.

Another exception is the unusual case where the aphasic difficulty strikes only one language area and leaves the others intact. This person may have no difficulty speaking, reading, or writing, but have great trouble understanding the speech of others. Or his difficulty may be limited to reading. Occasionally a patient will complain that he can write well but cannot read back what he has written. These are, in general, the kinds of aphasia where writing is not impaired or later recovers to its original status. Nearly all other aphasics continue to have writing problems permanently.

Aphasics who recover language well enough to return to work but were more than mildly impaired at onset, often find that writing causes them more difficulty than any other language skill. They may take such pains producing the finished product that no one else knows the struggle they have, but spelling and grammar may continue to present problems long after all other signs of aphasia have cleared.

Aphasic writing problems are frequently profound. Writing for most aphasics is often the most damaged language skill and the last to improve. When we consider that we learn to understand speech and to talk long before we read, and we learn to write after that, it is logical to view writing as among the highest and most complex symbolic language functions of human beings. Aphasics who can understand most of what is said, who have only a mild or moderate speech impairment, and who can read enough to get the gist of what is on a page, often can only produce a single written word now and then. They may be able to write a three letter word such as "tea" though it may often become "tee" or even "ten." They may start off correctly in a longer word and then become completely lost in a jumble of letters so that "football" becomes "foozdhltp."

Some aphasics cannot write words unless the words are dictated, because they cannot recall the word itself, but if they hear it spoken they have varying degrees of success with the spelling. Others have better luck if the words are slowly spelled to them, although aphasics who have lost the names of the letters will have even more problems when this is done.

Those who attempt to write sentences not only have trouble finding the words they want and spelling the words they use, but their grammar and syntax seem to have disintegrated. A sentence such as: "I want to see a movie" may be written as: "He seesh mofe," or a series of meaningless letters may be strung together such as "alfus arg wunch."

Interestingly enough, some patients write very painstakingly, producing only jumbled, meaningless letters, yet they seem to be so methodical in their attempts—even "reading" the "words" back silently—that it is clear they are not aware that their productions are meaningless. Others will not even attempt to write because they are fully aware that they cannot produce anything correctly. Many patients cannot write real letters at all, with most of their efforts resulting only in scribbles, the equivalent of meaningless jargon in speech.

Some aphasics can copy printed or written words well; others omit, reverse, or even substitute letters. Those whose eyes have trouble tracking may copy words or letters from above or below the line they are working on.

The size of the letters they are trying to copy is important. If they are having tracking and focusing problems, it is easier for them to copy larger print of perhaps a half inch in height than print of normal size used in books. Some aphasics have a condition called *constructional apraxia*. They have great difficulty figuring out how to copy an X or how to reproduce on paper geometric forms such as a square or triangle drawn within a circle. (These same patients will be unable to imitate various patterns made with colored blocks.) Since many letters have similar complexity to these geometric forms they will have little success trying to copy even the letters of the alphabet.

Is Writing Difficult Because He Has to Use His Unaccustomed Hand?

A large number of aphasic patients are paralyzed on the right side and are right-handed people, so they must learn to use their unaccustomed left hand for writing efforts as well as for eating, washing, shaving, combing hair, applying makeup, and other activities. There are a few people whose language centers are in the right rather than the left hemisphere of their brain, whose injury was to that side and whose paralysis, therefore, is on the left side of their bodies. These people were left-handed (although not all left handed people have right hemisphere language centers) and have the same difficulty that right-handed people do in learning to use their unaccustomed hand, the right one in this case. Early attempts to use the unparalyzed hand are usually awkward but with time and practice most aphasics learn to use it successfully. Having only one hand remains awkward for many tasks, but writing can be done with mechanical success after a while—providing the paper is secured so that the pen or pencil does not rotate or move it, thus making writing very difficult. Many aphasics develop a fine tremor in their "good" hand which appears whenever they try to write, although it may not be apparent at any other time.

There are two aspects of writing to consider when aphasic writing difficulties are discussed: (1) the mechanical, muscular aspect of handling the pen or pencil; and (2) the symbolic language aspect. The mechanical and muscular aspect was discussed above. There is no doubt that this presents great difficulties for many patients, but with time, good practice, and especially if they have the good fortune to be in an occupational therapy program designed to help them become proficient in activities of daily living (ADL), they can usually learn to do many things well with the unaccustomed hand—even produce legible writing or printing.

Aphasic writing difficulties, however, are not involved with mechanics; rather, they are apparent in the symbolic, linguistic aspects, the memory of the word itself, its meaning, its spelling, as well as the grammatical, syntactical structure of a sentence. Even if an aphasic patient is not paralyzed—and some are not—and can continue to use his accustomed hand, he will have these latter kinds of writing difficulties to the extent of his aphasic impairment.

If He Cannot Use Speech Effectively Is Writing a Good Substitute?

This question comes up so frequently that it appears necessary to deal with it separately, although the previous two sections may have made the answer obvious. Since in most cases of aphasia, writing is the most damaged language skill and the last to become functional, if it ever does, it is rare that writing can be used as an effective substitute for speech in an aphasic patient. When an aphasic cannot talk, but can write well enough to communicate what he wishes to express, it is likely that this patient has apraxia of speech rather than an aphasic speech impairment (Chapter X), or he has one of the unusual aphasic conditions described earlier in which speech is his only impaired language skill.

Someone with a very mild aphasia will often be able to use writing for communication although with impaired spelling and grammer. Those with moderate aphasia may be able to supplement their speech struggles with written words or parts of words they are trying to say, so that the listener is greatly aided in understanding what he wants to express. These patients should have paper and pencil nearby so their communicative efforts are made more effective by whatever writing they manage to produce.

The majority of aphasic patients cannot use writing effectively enough to permit its use as a substitute for speech, and regrettably, never will be able to use it this way.

If He Cannot Write, Is a Typewriter a Good Substitute?

This is another frequent question. In fact, many well-meaning family members or friends produce a typewriter triumphantly without consulting a speech pathologist, and are greatly disturbed when the patient has strong negative reactions to what they meant as a loving gesture. In the preceding sections it was made clear that if the patient has aphasia and therefore cannot write, he will not be able to find words, to spell, or to produce sentences any better with a typewriter than he can with a pen or pencil. In fact, the keyboard itself, with its display of letters, can produce such confusion that patients who can write a little with their good hand may become frustrated and anxious when facing a typewriter.

The patient who can use a typewriter well is most likely one who has little or no aphasia but a marked apraxia of speech, and who has no difficulty in visual tracking or in keeping his eyes in focus. Before presenting a typewriter to an aphasic patient it is best to discuss his condition with a speech pathologist who has tested his speech for apraxia, and who has accurate information about his writing ability.

Can Spelling Boards and Spelling Games Such as Scrabble and Crossword Puzzles Be of Help?

Families and friends, trying to be helpful, may bring these as gifts to the aphasic patient, who often becomes anxious by these offerings. The anxiety is produced by the feelings, as one patient later related to me, that if all these people expected him to be able to use these instruments, and he obviously could not, he must be in far worse shape than they realize. Not a comfortable conclusion for the patient who cannot even express his anxiety to someone able to explain that the choice of gift was an error in judgment on the part of the others—that his inability to use these devices was consistent with his condition.

When a patient has mild or no aphasia but has a severe apraxia of speech or a very severe dysarthria, he should be able to use a spelling board; but since he should also be able to write if he can spell, its use will probably be more cumbersome than pencil and paper. If he is someone whose paralysis includes both hands but who can move his fingers well enough to point to the letters he wants, he can be greatly benefitted by a spelling board since he may not be able to hold a pencil. But an aphasic patient will not very likely be able to use any of these instruments or games in any useful way, and it is unwise to present them to him without professional concurrence.

Can He Recover Ability to Spell and to Use Grammar and Syntax Correctly in Writing?

There appears to be a logical progression of recovery of various language skills in aphasia, consistent perhaps with the ways we first developed language in early childhood. Thus, understanding of speech is the first language area in most forms of aphasia to show signs of recovery and is usually the basic area of concern in therapy. Then speech itself begins to improve and to become more effective. Reading, in a very elementary form, may begin to emerge. But during these early days, writing is limited in most patients to copying only.

The person who cannot understand a word when it is said to him, who cannot verbally produce it himself regularly or at all, or who does not understand it when he tries to read it, will be most unlikely to be able to write the word. If he thinks and says "ickle" when he looks at a cup of coffee, he is apt to write a meaningless combination of letters for those words.

When an aphasic reaches a particular level of proficiency in understanding speech, speaking, reading, and using gestures meaningfully, he is sometimes spontaneously able to write words better than he has in the past, with enough correct letters so that others can understand more of what he is writing. With intensive writing therapy begun at that time he may continue to improve for a long time, even years after onset, but only a few ever recover to their previous writing capability. At this time there is no way to predict how far an individual patient who has begun to recover writing ability may progress, given adequate treatment. For many, however, it is obvious that treatment is futile and should not be attempted.

How Can He Be Helped to Improve Writing Ability?

Until he shows signs—through periodic aphasia testing—that he is beginning to write some words with fair success from dictation or spontaneously, the only writing he should be doing regularly is copying. Even this task must start at the level at which he begins to show evidence of problems. Therefore, if he cannot copy geometric forms or printed letters adequately, mastering ability to produce these through copying must precede any more complex tasks. He may always produce them with a tremor or distortions, but if the result is recognizable as the desired response, he can move on to another task.

When he can produce the letters correctly he may be given lists of words to copy. The paper he writes on should be fastened securely to the table top with scotch tape or to a heavy clip board, with the angle correct for his new need to use the unaccustomed hand. The words selected for him to copy are best placed where he will not conceal them by his writing arm. They should be words that will be important to him, especially his name if he is unable to write or print it without a model.

For most aphasics, copying is as far as they will ever progress in writing ability. Those who can procede will often need months of practice in writing from dictation before they can write the same words without this aid. After they can write the names of objects, of verbs, or prepositional phrases all describing pictures of these words, they may be ready to try short sentences. Each part of speech may need to be developed systematically. Grammar and syntax may only return dependably after years of effort and drill. Some will never become truly proficient but will get by. For many it will be wasted effort.

Chapter VIII

Aphasia: Gestures, Pantomime, and Signs

Can He Learn to Use Gestures, Pantomime, and
Signs?
Should the Use of Gestures Be Encouraged?
Should Gestures Be Used to the Aphasic Who Has Poor
Understanding of Speech?
How Can an Aphasic Learn to Use Gestures and
Pantomime?

Can He Learn to Use Gestures, Pantomime, and Signs?

We all normally use some forms of gestures, pantomime, and signing along
with speech. Many of these hand signals are universal or nearly so, such as
waving goodbye, nodding or shaking our heads to indicate yes or no,
hugging ourselves to show we are cold, waving a hand in front of our faces
with an audible breath to show we are too hot, and many more. In most
places of the world, regardless of language barriers, some of these signs and
gestures are well understood. Most of us are able to use forms of pantomime
to indicate certain activities if we want to communicate more intricate ideas
to others without speech. The parlor game "Charades" is based on this
ability. Of course, the professional mime has developed this faculty to a high
level art form, but most of us can do this at a simpler level capable of
informing others of our meaning without any accompanying words, if the
subject is not too abstract or complex. Most aphasics lose the ability to
communicate through these avenues to the same extent that they lose other
language skills.

Pantomime, gestures, and universal signs should be included in language
therapy with an aphasic for several important reasons. Primarily, if he can
recover some of this capacity, it will improve his ability to communicate when
he cannot find words to express his thoughts. Secondly, it has been found

that the use of gestures and signs, such as waving goodbye, helps some aphasics recover the word a gesture represents. It is a technique that has also been helpful with some patients who have apraxia of speech.

A third purpose is to help recover *symbolic* and *abstract ability* which are generally damaged in aphasia. Language itself is symbolic; a word is a symbol that takes the place of the object or the idea for which it stands. Gestures are also symbolic. Abstract ability is the human capacity to deal with theoretical, ideal, or general qualities, as opposed to *concrete ability* which deals with a particular thing or event. Brain injury often reduces or destroys ability to think in abstract terms and leaves the person with what is often referred to as *concrete thinking*. Recovering capacity to use gestures and to translate into pantomime certain ideas helps to stimulate abstract and symbolic ability in some patients, which in turn can improve language skills.

A fourth purpose is the value regaining these skills has for a particular group of patients who have certain forms of apraxia that prevent them from using their hands properly, although they are not paralyzed. These impairments are called *motor and sensory apraxia*. Those with motor apraxia have lost the ability to use an object properly, although they understand the nature and purpose of the object. This person may, for example, pick up a pair of scissors wanting to cut some thread, but he cannot recall what movements are necessary to make the scissors function properly. He will be likely to turn the scissors in all directions trying to find the right combination to make them work. *Sensory or ideational apraxia* prevents proper use of an object because the person has actually forgotten the object's nature and purpose. This patient will do such things as comb his hair with his toothbrush or try to drink his coffee with a knife. Some of these patients use the shower for a toilet or try to drink a dish of jello. Some patients with sensory apraxia have been diagnosed as demented, and indeed, if their behavior remains at this level with enough other intellectual impairments, they must be regarded as such. However, I have found that working through the gestural system with some of these patients has been an effective way to help them reorganize their perceptual and conceptual processes so that they can once again use objects properly.

Signs are common gestures shared by many people. Sign language, however, is an organized communication system that is taught to people who are deaf or who must communicate with deaf people. It is a complete language using the hands instead of the mouth for expressing ideas, and the eyes instead of ears for receiving them. As a general rule, an aphasic person cannot learn a new language, but can only hope to retrieve the language or languages he habitually used before his brain injury. Therefore, the only aphasic who can benefit from working with sign language is one who used it before he became aphasic. This person, if he is deaf and had no other way to communicate, will need to retrieve sign language in the same ways an aphasic hearing person must try to retrieve speech and the use of gestures.

Should the Use of Gestures Be Encouraged?

The goal of language therapy is to improve communication by any available means. A patient who can make his needs known through gestures should certainly be encouraged to do so.

A very valuable technique to help recover speech is to say aloud the word or words the gesture represents and to have the aphasic or apraxic person imitate that word while producing the gesture. Repeating these steps several or many times may stimulate the recovery of the word and its meaning permanently.

Should Gestures Be Used to the Aphasic Who Has Poor Understanding of Speech?

Whether or not gestures should be used along with words when speaking to an aphasic depends upon the situation and what the immediate goal is. If the need is to have him understand what is being said as well as he is able, it is necessary to use every avenue available to get the meaning across to him.

In social situations and in daily communication every effort should be made to help him understand and participate as fully as possible in the conversation going on around him. This means, of course, using any measures effective to aid in his comprehension—gestures, writing, pantomime, pictures, drawings, "pidgeon English"—anything that might work. If, however, the goal is to learn how well he understands speech without any cues or other embellishments, then it is important to avoid using any clue that might betray the meaning other than the words themselves. This means that hands must not move and eyes must look directly into his, remaining neutral in expression. Facial and body movements must be well controlled. Aphasics often become very sensitive to extremely small movements, gestures, or expressions, so when it is necessary to know what he understands of speech alone, other non-speech ways of conveying meaning must be avoided.

When attempting to help him to understand speech better in therapy or home treatment, words should be used alone without any gestural accompaniment, except if needed initially to help him understand what is wanted of him (see Chapter IV).

How Can an Aphasic Learn to Use Gestures and Pantomime?

A group of objects may be placed before the patient and he may be asked to demonstrate how each is used. It is usually necessary to show the patient the response that is wanted, because many aphasics do not understand what is being asked of them. When he starts to comply he should be dissuaded from talking during the action. The ultimate goal is for him to pretend to use the item as completely as if he were actually using it for the purpose it serves. Thus, a soup spoon would be tilted to pick up soup and then carried to his mouth. he should then act as if he were swallowing the liquid before the act is called complete. Merely picking up the spoon and waving it vaguely toward his mouth is not good enough, yet this is what many aphasics will do, sometimes for months, sometimes permanently.

When he usually gives a good performance with eight or ten items, the next step is to remove the item itself and have him pretend to be using it, performing just as he did with the actual object. It may be necessary to show him the object first, or a picture of it, if he does not understand the word for it reliably. If he is to learn to use pantomime effectively in order to express what he wants without speech, he must be able to go through the actions without the object, and to get the point across to someone who can interpret his meaning. Many aphasics love to do this and become very proficient at it, with dramatic embellishments and nicely conceived complexities. These people become well tuned in to the world around them, as a general rule, although still aphasic or apraxic of speech.

Finally, he must select an act he wants to present in pantomime, and others must interpret correctly what he means. Only then can he hope to use pantomime successfully to replace speech.

Chapter IX

Aphasia: Numbers, Arithmetic, and Time

Does He Know the Names of Numbers? Can He Count?
Does His Calculation Ability Seem Intact?
If He Passes All Tests of Calculation Ability, Should He
 Be Presumed Safe to Handle Financial Matters?
What Should Be Done When He Insists upon Resuming
 Financial Responsibility Although He Has Problems
 with Calculations?
Can He Improve Ability with Numbers and Calcula-
 tions?
Is Card Playing Affected by Loss of Calculation Ability?
Is His Knowledge of Time Intact?
How Can He Be Helped to Improve His Abilities with
 Numbers, Arithmetic, and Time?

Does He Know the Names of Numbers? Can He Count?

Some aphasics have as much trouble with numbers, arithmetic, and time as they do with any other language skill. Arithmetic is a form of language, a fact that surprises many people. Numbers are highly symbolic, just as words are, each number standing for a real idea as a word does. We do not have to write apple eight times because we can write "8 apples." We calculate and make extremely complex computations and tell time and keep in touch with calendar dates all with the use of numbers. In evaluating an aphasic's language status, his number, arithmetic, and time concepts must also be investigated, and it is good to start with his ability to count, to recognize numbers, and to say their names correctly.

There are many variations of difficulties with numbers, and it is easy to overlook serious deficiencies in this area by not understanding what to look for. An aphasic may be able to count by rote correctly yet have no idea what counting means, so that if he is asked how many there are of a particular item, he may be completely unable to deal with that concept. Another patient may understand that a number is wanted, and actually count the items as he should, but be unable to isolate the final number reached as the amount of that particular item. The concept of counting in relation to amount is impaired.

A patient may see a list of numbers and read or say them incorrectly, yet have a good number concept. For example, he may point to the number nine and call it seven, yet be able to place the number nine on a row of nine buttons. Others may have lost all of this basic ability. Some aphasics can name numbers correctly when they read them and also retain the concept the number represents, yet have no abiity to calculate.

The patient who can count well but has no concept of the meaning of counting has retained a long learned, rote skill; however, he may not only have lost the concept of amount, but also the names of the numbers except in this rote situation. As in all aphasia, many patients are inconsistent and tend to fluctuate in their adequacy with numbers.

The aphasic should be asked to count to 10; if he does that well then he may count up to 50 or 100, and any errors noted. Counting objects and presenting the total of those objects is another step. He may count to five well but when asked to tell how many there are of five pencils, he may be puzzled and frustrated. Then a list of numbers should be presented and he should be asked to point to each as it is randomly named by the examiner. Groups of objects arranged in sets of twos, threes, fours, etc., can be placed before him, and he may be asked to point to the group containing two, four, and so on. If he does that well, then he might be asked to place a card bearing a number on the group it represents. He might then be required to read the name of each number aloud depending upon his verbal ability, with care taken by the examiner not to have the numbers in the order of rote counting. Even if he made errors in any or all of these steps, calculation ability should be checked, because some aphasics have lost the names and concepts of numbers in one set of numerical tasks but have retained ability to use numbers well in other situations.

Does His Calculation Ability Seem Intact?

The patient's ability to calculate is fairly easy to check. A page of very simple arithmetic problems is given, starting at single number addition levels, such as 2 + 1, 3 + 4, 6 + 6, etc. The difficulty should only be increased as his competency in computing these basic figures is verified. A recheck should be made of all of his responses on another day in order to determine if he fluctuates in adequacy.

Even a mildly aphasic patient may have arithmetic impairment. On the other hand, some patients, even with moderate aphasia, retain calculation ability with no sign of any difficulty. It would be a rare event, however, to find a severely impaired aphasic patient who is able to use numbers in any meaningful way and who retains ability to calculate.

If He Passes All Tests of Calculation Ability, Should He Be Presumed Safe to Handle Financial Matters?

Anyone who has suffered brain injury, no matter how mild or how fully he appears to have recovered all his former abilities, may have some occasional difficulty with numbers and with calculation. Trouble may only occur when he is tired or under stress or have too many things to attend at one time, but it can occur. If the patient, his employer, and family are alert to this possibility, he might be advised to have someone check his figures when he is experiencing any of these conditions, rather than risk potentially serious consequences. Since many people who have not suffered brain injury have problems with arithmetic, especially when tired, stressed, or overloaded with stimuli, it need not be a threat to the patient's ego to have a safeguard against error, unless perhaps if he is an accountant or someone who has always handled numbers exceedingly well.

A patient of mine was a C.P.A. who felt he could go on with his business when he recovered from his stroke. He appeared to have retained all his calculation skills, but I had strong misgivings about his ability to handle clients' accounts during the approaching stressful income tax season. I had discussed this with him and with his wife, but he was adamant to return to his practice, terminating therapy. His wife called me sometime later with the unhappy news that he had indeed found the entire scene to be too overwhelming, and had turned his practice over to his partner. He had found himself reaching recurring blocks when he was fatigued, which he often was during those weeks, and would stare at the pages of returns for hours, unable to figure out how to begin. It was fortunate for his clients that he recognized his inability to perform under these circumstances and withdrew before he could make a shambles of anyone's returns.

What Should Be Done When He Insists Upon Resuming Financial Responsibility Although He Has Problems with Calculations?

Some wives are reluctant to interfere when their husbands wish to take over the family or business finances, even though they realize their husbands are not performing at former levels of competency in arithmetic and numerical concepts. In some cases they are hesitant because they feel that to do so will rob their husbands of their "masculine role" as head of household; in others they fear that warning the firm's management about the calculation risk might jeopardize the job. They appear to behave much like the proverbial ostrich, hoping that by keeping their heads in the sand, not facing the issue, it will go away and all will be well. It rarely works that way. Sooner or later, trouble will strike.

The aphasic who has obvious impairment of these functions does not have the opportunity to makes these kinds of often disasterous choices. It is the patient who is on the borderline, who can perform correctly enough at times that others can be lulled into thinking he does as well as ever, who gets into these unfortunate situations. He may write checks correctly nine out of ten times, but the tenth check may be for $2000.00 when he meant $200.00. Or he might order 1,000,000 pencils when he intended to order 1000. He can make enough errors in calculation to mess up the business' books or to overdraw the family's bank account seriously.

It is important to deal with reality, and reality dictates honest appraisal of residual problems. Sometimes all it means is that he can assume all his former responsibilities but someone must be alerted to check his results before they are acted upon. In this way he can learn what his errors are and work on them, if possible. With enough work he may overcome the problem, but if a pretence of no difficulty is maintained, there is little chance that he will attempt to overcome the problem. Reality may also mean that he must give up former responsibilities of check writing, placing orders, keeping books, etc. He may have to go through a period of depression and anger over this loss, but brain injury nearly always requires relinquishing some accustomed form of life-style. A sensitive, empathetic family can look for ways to restore his feelings of self worth that will not endanger the family's economic structure nor that of a business.

The wife of a patient of mine found a solution that worked well for them. Her husband wanted to deal with real money, not just therapy problems. She contacted their bank and discussed the problem her husband had with figures, telling that he wanted practice writing checks and balancing his checkbook, but had agreed that he made too many errors to take the entire responsibility. She also alerted shopkeepers with whom he was most likely to do business. He was working hard on his arithmetic in therapy and at home and was encouraged, as we all were, by his steady improvement, but he still made errors in calculation and his checkbook had to be rebalanced frequently. His errors were used as therapy material. A small account was opened for him and he understood that he was in charge of only a miniscule amount of the family's resources, but this gave him a great feeling of building toward a goal. If he had been denied any contact with the handling of money he would have felt quite impotent, although for many patients that is the only solution. For most patients it is better to use a check book in which to practice without a real bank account backing it up. The patient might write checks without using them for all situations that require checks, and balance the stubs himself each time. Only when, after weeks or months of this simulated activity, it becomes clear that he is well able to assume this function, need it become a reality. His errors during this period can become therapy material.

Can He Improve Ability with Numbers and Calculation?

As in all language skills, it is possible for many patients to improve in this area also, and some will need long months of concentrated work to reach their ultimate potential. The difference between working with arithmetic and working in other language areas is that communication improvement is the goal of the latter and for that, one does not have to recover former exactness of syntax, grammar, or even the selection of the better word. In calculation, of course, there is only one choice and that is the correct one. Most aphasics who lose some ability to calculate will never recover it to their former levels of competence. It then becomes a matter of choice to decide how much time and effort should be expended in this area. "Ultimate potential" does not necessarily mean what the patient wants it to mean. There will come a time when, no matter how much concentration he brings to bear on figures, he will not be able to improve beyond that. There is no way to predict that level at this time, and if it falls short of his previous ability, that will have to become acceptable.

People whose life-style does not require them to use calculations, and particularly those who do not wish to cope with them, need not be troubled with arithmetic in therapy. All patients who are not severely aphasic should be screened to determine their number and arithmetic ability, but whether a therapy program is initiated depends upon results of the screening and upon the patient's and therapist's decisions. A patient may unrealistically wish to pursue this avenue, and the therapist may realize that he is not able to function well enough to begin such a program. He must be told he is not ready and perhaps sometime later arithmetic work can be started.

All testing results should be carefully dated and retained. If after several months of effort documentation reveals that there is no change, it is probably best to drop the program, at least for that period of time. Perhaps in six more months or later he might be better able to profit from work in these areas. It may be that as his other language areas improve, ability to profit from arithmetic work will improve also. This occurs with some aphasics in reading and writing, so it may well occur with arithmetic also. Documentation serves the added purpose of reassuring a patient that in the recent period of time he has improved. It is very encouraging for the patient to be shown evidence that six months earlier he could not add $8 + 2$ and now he is correctly adding figures such as $89 + 24$.

Is Card Playing Affected by Loss of Calculation Ability?

Some aphasics who cannot talk well or calculate perfectly have retained an astonishing ability to play well whatever card games they enjoyed before the brain injury occurred. Some may be unable to keep score or even to say "gin" or to name the cards, but have no difficulty playing the game. If card playing was an important part of the patient's life, he should be tested to determine if he can still play, because it can certainly enhance the quality of his life if he can continue to enjoy this activity.

Is His Knowledge of Time Intact?

Some aphasics can tell time very accurately. Others are totally unable to deal with time at any level. Between these two extremes are a variety of difficulties.

Some who tell time accurately may be unable to say the words, read the numbers when not on a clock, or to write them. Some can recognize the hour or even the half-hour, but are unable to understand the minutes in between these times. Some may appear to understand well and even say the times correctly aloud, but either recall them poorly later or confuse them in some way. For example, a patient may make an appointment for 9 AM all the while thinking 2 PM, and therefore show up at the later time. Another aphasic may think someone was coming home at 2 PM and become quite disturbed when that person did not appear until 4 PM, the actual stated time for arrival.

The husband of an aphasic patient was unaware that his wife could not tell time or make much sense out of numbers. Before she started speech therapy she had been able to resume cooking at home, and usually did well, except that she never seemed to put roasts into the oven on time or set the oven at the correct temperature. After her number and time concepts were tested and found to be defective, he understood her problem and was able to find a solution so he could come home to a properly prepared meal. It required his cooperation and planning ahead. When they were having an oven cooked meal he would set the control at the correct temperature before he left for work in the morning, calling her later when it was time to turn the oven on for preheating. Those people who have automatic ovens can work this out more easily.

To check some aspects of an aphasic's ability to tell time, a clock should be used along with times written on paper, such as 9:00, 12:30, or 2:45. As the clock is set to one of these he is asked to point to the corresponding number on the paper. Then, without the clock, the examiner may say aloud each of the times on the paper and the patient must point to it. There are patients who have a fine sense of time, but do not know the names of the numbers when they are spoken to them, so they will be unable to point corectly to 9:00 when it is spoken yet show up promptly for a 9 o'clock appointment, because it was written down for them.

Testing all aspects of a patient's potential problems with time is very difficult. Only experience may reveal certain confusions, especially when they fluctuate in adequacy. It is necessary, therefore, for those who are in contact with aphasics to realize that when time is involved in a patient's performance and that performance is faulty, a confusion concerning time may have been the cause, rather than some other kind of difficulty.

The day, the month, and the year are easily forgotten by a hospitalized patient, even without aphasia. Many hospitals now are clearly posting this information where patients can see it daily. The aphasic patient who does not read the newspapers, or who has problems understanding written or spoken words, can very well lose all sense of time in relation to the day, the month, or the year. This was dramatically revealed to me when I was a student working with an aphasic patient who had been in a nursing home for years and was at last receiving speech therapy he could have benefitted from years earlier. At one point he mentioned his age, stating it as five years younger than he actually was. He knew the day and month, but had lost track of the years and actually believed this to be five years earlier. In my naiveté as an inexperienced student, I hastened to correct his error and he had what is often referred to as a "castastrophic reaction," the only one I have ever seen in all my years of working with aphasic patients. This term describes a violent emotional blow-up that brain injured people are supposedly prone to; in my experience, however, it is not as likely to happen as students are often led to believe. Perhaps that early exprience prepared me to anticipate and protect against them, for it was a profoundly disturbing occurrence for both of us. Whether or not an aphasic can read or understand, he should have daily access to the printed and spoken information of the fully presented date. There are so many subtle and little known ways through which aphasics may obtain information, that this knowledge should be presented to him regularly, on the chance that some of it may get through to him. Keeping in touch with time is an important way to keep in touch with reality. Making an issue of his birthday celebration each year can be an important and pleasant way to keep him in touch with time and his age.

How Can He Be Helped to Improve His Abilities with Numbers, Arithmetic, and Time?

If it is determined that he may benefit from time spent working in this area, the first important information to obtain is exactly at what level he begins to have problems. It is very necessary to work at that level and not beyond it, because only where he begins to make errors is he accessible to improvement. A patient who is making errors adding such figures as 24 + 63 should not be given problems involving the carrying of even one number. Well-meaning family members who are untrained but eager, often tend to work far beyond the patient's level of ability, usually for fear of insulting his intelligence if they present problems at a lower but more realistic level. Unless a patient has success with at least 90 percent of the problems presented to him at any level, he is clearly not ready to work there. Even with 90 percent success, he still needs much drill at the lower level to prepare him for greater success here. Before he succeeds with 100 percent of the problems, he should not move on. Arithmetic needs to be correct 100 percent of the time before it can be useful in real life situations.

Chapter X

Apraxia of Speech and Oral Apraxia

What Is Apraxia of Speech?
What Is Oral Apraxia?
When Should Apraxia Therapy Be Started?
Is a Speech Pathologist Necessary to Treat Apraxia of Speech?
Does Apraxia Ever Improve Long After Onset?
How Can Others Help in Treatment of Apraxia?
Can an Apraxic Patient Be Helped to Communicate in Other Ways?

What Is Apraxia of Speech?

Apraxia of speech is the inability to produce a word, phrase, or sentence voluntarily because the apraxic patient cannot recall how to place his tongue, lips, and other parts of the speech production mechanism in the correct positions to form speech sounds and to sequence these sounds in the proper order to make desired words. Apraxia of speech, although it is limited to speech, does not involve the linguistic, symbolic aspect of language as does aphasia. The apraxic patient may well know the word he wants to say and the meaning of that word, but he has great difficulty, often even total failure, uttering it, not just when he tries to say it without a model, but in imitating someone else's utterance of the word. Although apraxia is a mechanical problem involving the muscles used to produce speech, it is not a result of weakness or paralysis of these muscles as in dysarthria. The patient can be observed using all these same muscles adequately for chewing, swallowing, licking his lips, raising his tongue, and even, perhaps, saying the same words automatically that he fails to say volitionally.

Apraxia of speech does not usually exist alone without aphasia, because the injury producing apraxia also often causes aphasia. In many cases this same patient has dysarthria as well. When all three of these conditions occur together, it is very difficult to determine the extent of each, but it is important to do so as much as possible because each requires a very different treatment from the other.

Some severely apraxic patients can only utter such sounds as "dee dee dee" or perhaps a single word such as "hello," which they use for every verbal attempt. Some can only produce profanities or a four-letter word that emerges in every speech attempt. One hospital patient could only say "fire, fire, fire" which he often emitted in full voice, much to the consternation of the other patients and hospital staff.

Until recent years speech pathologists along with physicians called apraxia of speech "expressive aphasia," not distinguishing it from the word-finding, aphasic level of difficulty. Because it was wrongly viewed as part of the symbolic language problem it was treated as such, and therapy usually failed. When speech pathologists began to treat it as a problem separate from aphasia and developed different approaches to its treatment, exciting breakthroughs began to occur. This is not to imply that a severely apraxic patient is ever likely to become a fluent speaker, but many who are now able to speak a word or phrase, to express a need or a thought, formerly would never have been able to communicate these ideas.

An aphasic patient who has no apraxia or dysarthria should have no difficulty imitating a word or a phrase spoken to him, providing he understands what he is being asked to do. In order to make the proper diagnosis, it is important that the patient really is aware of what is wanted, and that his failure to imitate is not due to poor comprehension. When there is reason to suspect the latter, gestures may be needed to make him understand. Placing a mirror before him and the examiner, who points to his own mouth as he says a short word, and then to the patient's mouth indicating he wants the same response, may sometimes help the patient understand what is wanted. An aphasic patient can imitate a word even if he does not recall its meaning.

The patient who has dysarthria will not be able to produce certain sounds well or at all because the muscles needed to make these sounds cannot move the lips, tongue, or other parts of the speech mechanism into the proper positions. If a patient cannot raise his tongue tip, for example, to lick peanut butter or jelly from the roof of his mouth, he will not be able to produce correctly the sounds "l," "t," "d," and "n," and certain other sounds may be distorted. If this patient also has apraxia of speech, he will of course, be unable to imitate correctly words containing these sounds, even though he eventually learns to imitate other words well. A careful assessment must be made by the examiner of how much of his failure is due to the paralysis and how much to the apraxia. When dysarthria is found to exist along with suspected apraxia, a full analysis of the sounds affected by the paralysis must be made. These need to be avoided when an apraxia text is given, and should not be used in apraxia treatment unless the patient becomes very proficient at imitation and volitional production of other words.

Apraxia of speech may be mild. If the aphasia is also mild these are the patients who can say many words and even attempt sentences, but with many mispronunciations as they keep aiming for the target over and over. They may sound exactly like a dysarthric at times, but unlike that patient, they are capable of making the sounds entirely correctly, perhaps on the next try. They may sound like an aphasic who is not apraxic, because they may appear to be hunting for a word, rather than the pronunciation of that word.

Apraxics may be able to imitate words well but break down when trying to imitate phrases or short sentences. This may be due to apraxic sequencing problems that appear when the task becomes more complex, or it may be due to a reduced auditory retention span. If a patient cannot keep a model in mind that has more than two or three elements, he will have great difficulty imitating a phrase containing more individual units than this. When a patient reveals difficulty imitating longer material, it is advisable to check his auditory memory span before going on with more apraxia therapy (Chapter II). If his memory cannot be improved, the number of units presented to him for imitation must be kept within the boundaries of his ability to recall.

The apraxic patient who is not aphasic or whose aphasia is such that he is able to write well, will be able to write those words or sentences that he cannot say. There are times when the ability to write helps in the diagnosis of apraxia. When it is unclear whether a patient is not able to produce a word because he cannot recall the name of the object or because he cannot place his mouth and tongue in the correct positions to produce that word, his ability to write it often helps the examiner understand the nature of the problem. Of course, there are exceptions, such as patients who may write well but have verbal aphasic word-finding difficulties.

Some speech pathologists refer to apraxia of speech as oral verbal apraxia; others call it verbal apraxia. These terms all refer to the same condition, different from *oral apraxia*.

What Is Oral Apraxia?

Oral apraxia means an inability to move volitionally any of the oral muscles although they can all move normally for eating, swallowing, yawning, sucking, blowing, and so on, when these acts are carried out as routine functions, not as imitative or volitional acts. The difference between this and apraxia of speech is that oral apraxia does not involve speech sounds or words. The orally apraxic patient will have difficulty following commands to stick out his tongue, purse his lips, pull the lips back into a smile, even when it is clear that he understands what he is told to do. He will have little or no more success imitating these movements. In trying to stick out his tongue he might be seen to pull it back, or the tip will rise or remain rigidly on the floor of the mouth. His brain is not sending the correct signals to the muscles to tell them what to do to perform the task properly. It is necessary to rule out dysarthria as the cause, and this is done by observing how well he makes these same movements when not specifically trying to do so but with some other goal in mind. When a patient is seen to lick jelly off his lips in a normal sequence of movements, but is unable to move his tongue from side to side across his lips when told to do so, dysarthria cannot be considered as the cause of the problem. This is instead due to oral apraxia.

Oral apraxia and apraxia of speech do not necessarily exist together; a patient may have one without the other. If a patient has oral apraxia but no apraxia of speech, he should not have any significant interference with speech production. If he has both, I have not always found it necessary to work with the oral apraxia before attempting to treat the apraxia of speech. However, if his apraxia of speech is so profound that he cannot produce voice or cannot begin to make an attempt at imitating a speech sound, it may be necessary to start at the more primitive levels of imitating mouth and tongue movements, breathing movements, production of sighs, blowing, etc., before attempting to work with speech sounds or word imitation.

When Should Apraxia Therapy Be Started?

Apraxia of speech, unlike aphasia, does not have a timetable of improvement for the first six months after stroke, nor does it usually improve without treatment regardless of cause, as aphasia generally does for a time. Only when the cause is a completely reversible condition that leaves little or no residual damage when it resolves, does apraxia improve or clear up without therapy. These reversible conditions include brain hemorrhage, severe edema, hydrocephalus, and brain tumor. Under some circumstances, when these are resolved, patients may return to normal functioning. A patient with apraxia of speech who does not have a reversible condition as the cause will rarely be able to regain much voluntary control of his speech-producing mechanism without special help. Even with intensive apraxia therapy, it may take a long time to make any headway at all, if ever.

Because of the difficulty of treating apraxia, I prefer to begin apraxia therapy as soon as the patient's physician pronounces him strong enough to start therapy—even the first week following stroke. The aphasic patient should be tested with a comprehensive aphasia test before aphasia therapy is begun, and this is best given at one month after onset of stroke, or whenever he has stabilized after other causes. The apraxic patient needs only a diagnosis of apraxia, as opposed to aphasic word-finding problems or dysarthric impairment, in order for therapy to begin. Left untreated he will most likely remain unable to utter more than a "dee dee dee" or other automatic phrase, or to struggle with many false starts until he approaches his target. The voiceless apraxic patient may very well never produce voice voluntarily without special help.

The apraxic patient, as well as the aphasic, may be very frightened by his speech problem, and therapy can do much for both to offer encouragement that help is at hand. However, the untreated aphasic who is improving spontaneously receives encouragement from this experience, whereas the apraxic patient is unlikely to have this happen. His fear generally intensifies as time goes on and he cannot speak better if no one is trying to help him.

Is a Speech Therapist Necessary to Treat Apraxia of Speech?

Therapy for apraxia often involves techniques that people untrained in speech pathology cannot possible be aware of unless they are in touch with speech pathologists who can guide them in a home program. There are a variety of approaches to the treatment of apraxia. What works with one patient may not work with another. A knowledge of many different methods is especially helpful so that they can be tried, combined, eliminated, and modified as results of their use are noted. It appears to be far more difficult to start the process of speech production in an apraxic patient than it is to start the process of word finding in an aphasic patient.

Some speech pathologists are conducting research into different and effective ways of treating apraxia. They share their results with colleagues through professional journals, workshops, and meetings. Some of these techniques include use of singing long known songs, of a type of melodic chanting, of a systematic series of steps of mutual participation between patient and therapist where sounds or words are presented, spoken in unison, then alone and in various combinations. Use of a mirror is a fine method with some apraxics but very inhibiting to others. Building words from individual speech sounds is the best approach for some, valueless for others. Icing of the oral muscles in particular ways is dramatically effective for some apraxics, whereas for others it is a waste of time. Recently an apraxic patient of mine experienced production of his first word immediately following the application of ice to his mouth, tongue, lips, and cheeks for the first time. He had for weeks made no progress whatsoever until icing was tried. Since that time he has learned to say a number of words and is now producing short sentences. All of these have had to be taught as he has not yet experienced spontaneous production of any words. Some apraxics do well in groups with other apraxic patients; some only do well working alone with the therapist.

Without contact with a speech pathologist experienced in apraxia therapy, home treatment is usually of no value. Professional guidance is necessary, at least until techniques are found that are effective with a particular patient and whose family is well trained to continue the methods at home. Even then it is important to check with the therapist at arranged times for further guidance, because new approaches usually become necessary after a while in order for the patient to make further progress.

Does Apraxia Ever Improve Long After Onset?

Apraxic patients who have good understanding of speech and little or no dysarthria often are able to learn to say many words, short phrases, and sentences, continuing to add these to their ever increasing repertoire for years after onset. Patients who have never received apraxia therapy and who start it even six or more years later can make surprising progress, very gratifying to them and to their families. These same patients obviously made no progress without professional treatment because the families usually tried to help them at home, to no purpose.

Patients who are severely aphasic as well as apraxic, or who have a profound inability to understand speech and to monitor their own speech, are very poor candidates for apraxia therapy. Unless their aphasia improves with time so that they understand and self-monitor much better, there is no purpose in attempting apraxia therapy at a later date.

Dysarthric patients who also have apraxia may benefit from apraxia therapy for a long period of time, providing the dysarthria is not so severe that few speech sounds can be successfully produced. In that case, apraxia therapy is of no value.

There are many patients who, once they regain the process of speaking at will, begin to add words spontaneously that have not been painstakingly taught in therapy. Many other patients, however, never produce any speech that has not been presented in the therapy hour and worked over with great effort before it becomes habitual. Regardless of how they regain some speech or how long it takes, I have never known a severely apraxic patient to become proficient in speech production to the point where he could be called a fluent speaker. Many, at best, may be able to say such sentences as: "I am sad" or "I am happy," having learned these phrases in therapy. They may use one or two words appropriately to signify what they want to say, and with the questions put to them by the listener, be able to make their meaning clear at last. They may use synonyms or a related word, such as "lemons" when they mean "oranges," because they learned to say "lemons" but never mastered the word "oranges."

A patient may suddenly have a breakthrough because of a new approach, even years after therapy began. Recently a patient of mine who had to leave therapy three years earlier, returned to treatment eight years after onset, with his apraxia, although still severe, quite notably improved from when I had seen him last. Naturally I investigated to find what had caused this fine improvement. I learned that no one had been working with him but he had been regularly watching "Sesame Street" daily for the last year or two, imitating the speech sounds and words they use in speech games on that program. His ability to imitate had improved before leaving therapy, but now it was excellent and the stimulus of the individual words presented on that show, repeated over and over as they do, was exactly what he needed to make many of these words habitual. He had added more than 50 words to his vocabulary during those years. Back in treatment now, he has been able to build phrases and short sentences with these words as a base, and he continues to improve all these years after onset.

Help can come in unexpected ways. I would never have thought to suggest a program like "Sesame Street" to an adult, because many adults would find this very threatening. They would view this as an admission that they have been reduced to childhood levels in their mental functioning. Yet this patient found the program to be of great help, and it is possible that many other patients can also, if they overcome their fear of what it implies.

How Can Others Help in Treatment of Apraxia?

Family, friends, and ward personnel can be of great help in reinforcing what the speech pathologist is working on in therapy. When a patient's newly acquired word is reinforced throughout the day by many who come in contact with him, that word has a better chance of becoming habitual than if it is only used in the therapy hour a few times a week. For example, if he has finally been able to say the word "coffee" at will with the therapist, but never uses it outside of treatment, it may not emerge to become useful. If, however, his wife has been taught how to stimulate the word, and by attending his therapy sessions knows that he has acquired it and now reinforces it at home, he has a very good chance of making that word a useful one for him. To reinforce it, she would insist that he always say the word to her before he receives a cup of coffee, and perhaps see that he says it once or twice while he drinks it.

The apraxic patient is usually very slow in producing the words he has learned to say, so it is necessary that others allow him to have ample time to frame the words he tries to utter. On the other hand, an apraxic must not be permitted to take long periods of time when it is known that he seldom produces any words successfully. Apraxic patients can become conditioned to remain at the center of attention for long periods without any productive communication emerging if steps are not taken to prevent this. Regrets may be expressed by others that they cannot understand the patient at this time, stating that sometime later he may be able to say the word he wants, especially if he works hard in therapy.

The wife of a patient, some weeks after her husband was released from the hospital, expressed the fact that she was exhausted because she had so little time to do her chores, needing to spend so much time trying to understand what he wanted to say to her, and usually failing at this. When it was made clear to her that she must only try for a few moments, because he had not yet reached the point in apraxia therapy where he could produce a meaningful word at will, her home life became more tolerable and she found ample time to complete her chores. By attending therapy, she knew when he was able to say a particular word, and made certain he had ample time to produce that word at home.

Can an Apraxic Patient Be Helped to Communicate in Other Ways?

The apraxic patient whose aphasia is so mild that he can write well enough to express himself has this avenue through which he can communicate. He should always have with him a notebook or magic slate, the kind used by children from which words disappear when the plastic cover is raised. Many aphasic-apraxic patients cannot write, of course—nor will they ever be able to—so other means need to be found to help them express their thoughts very early after onset, while apraxia therapy is going on.

If the apraxic's gestures are intelligible, he must be encouraged to use them as much as possible. Gestures, however, are limited, even when intact. Since brain injured people often have damage to their gestural capacity, many apraxic patients have very reduced ability to communicate effectively through this means. Systematic therapy with gestural language helps some patients communicate to a certain extent through gestures (Chapter VIII).

If he can read, a notebook arrangement of words he is apt to use frequently is sometimes an effective tool. He might carry a small dictionary with him at all times, and point to the words he cannot say. This, of course, means that his listener takes ample time to be with him while he finds the correct words, and then reads the ones he points to in the book.

A communication notebook with pictures of objects and of the people most important in his life should be provided for him as early as possible, if he cannot read.

A spelling board is only beneficial to a patient who cannot use his hands for writing but is able to spell the words he wants to say by pointing to each letter. Obviously, if he can write, it is more efficient to do so than to point laboriously to individual letters. Paralysis that prevents writing may also prevent pointing, however.

Some patients are able to draw well enough to convey their meaning, although I must admit that I have found few patients who are able to use this means effectively.

It is very challenging to find ways through which an apraxic can communicate with little or no speech. For those with multiple aphasic problems as well, it may be impossible to find any reliable avenue through which they can make their meaning clear. As with aphasics, no one should pretend to understand what an apraxic is trying to express when the meaning is obscure or unknown. It is good to state to an apraxic what the listener believes he is trying to say, if he has a clue, and ask if that is his meaning. Sometimes, by the process of elimination and use of trial and error, his thoughts finally become evident. All of this takes time, and after warning that an apraxic must not be permitted to take up long periods of time unproductively, this may sound contradictory. However, the apraxic patient who has no one around who is willing to take time with him while he works out what he wants to say, will very often give up trying and withdraw into noncommunicating silence and depression. To achieve a good balance the listener needs to know how productive an apraxic's efforts are likely to be and how much time he requires generally to reach his goal. This much time should be allowed. The patient who rarely manages to convey his meaning after five or more minutes is the one who must not be permitted to hold the floor indefinitely.

Chapter XI

Dysarthria

What Is Dysarthria?
Is a Speech Therapist Necessary to Treat Dysarthria?
Can a Layman Help Him to Speak More Clearly?
How Can Ice Be Used to Help Some Forms of Dysarthria?
Does Dysarthria Ever Improve Long After Onset?

What Is Dysarthria?

Dysarthria is an impairment of speech or voice caused by brain injury and resulting in weakness or paralysis of muscles that are used to produce speech and voice. Total paralysis of these muscles results in death, because many of these are the same muscles needed for breathing and swallowing; therefore, in dysarthria, there are always enough muscles functioning to assure survival.

When muscles needed for swallowing are impaired, the patient may have to be fed through a tube. He may drool a great deal because he cannot readily swallow his saliva. If the vocal cords are partially paralyzed or weak, his voice will be hoarse or very soft, even just a whisper. A whispered or very weak voice can also result when the muscles of the abdomen, the diaphragm, or the chest are weakened because these are needed to set the vocal cords into vibration in order to produce a normally strong voice. When the muscles at the back of the mouth and throat are affected, the voice will be very nasal, because these are the muscles that close off the nasal passage and prevent the voice from emerging through the nose. When voice goes through the nasal passage it becomes nasalized. In English we have only three nasal speech sounds, m, n, and ng. Nasalizing other speech sounds often results in poor intelligibility. People with this problem have difficulty pronouncing the sounds k and hard g, among others, so that words like "cake" and "go" become very difficulty to understand. When the muscles of the tongue, cheeks, and lips are affected many speech sounds become distorted, completely altered, or cannot be produced at all.

Dysarthria ranges from very mild, so that a patient sounds a bit different from the way he habitually talked but can be well understood, through varying degrees of poorer intelligibility, to a total inability to speak a single word that can be understood although he may not be aphasic or apraxic at all. Of course, if dysarthria exists along with either or both of these conditions, the problems are more severe.

Is a Speech Therapist Necessary to Treat Dysarthria?

A speech therapist should be consulted to determine if there are any ways the patient's speech can be made more intelligible. In some cases, intact muscles are not being used by the patient fully because the surrounding muscles are so weakened that it takes too much effort to put the good muscles into movement. The same sort of thing happens when muscles in other parts of the body become paralyzed or weakened. The tendency is to stop using, or not use fully, muscles that still have ability to function. Many people can learn to walk again or use a partially paralyzed arm or hand after working with a physical therapist. If paralysis is total in a muscle there is no way to revive it because its control center in the brain has been destroyed. It is the surrounding muscles that may be put to better use in any course of therapy offered by physical and occupational therapists. With better use of the muscles needed to produce speech, intelligibility will be improved. A speech pathologist experienced in the diagnosis and treatment of dysarthria should be consulted to make the determination of whether or not treatment might help.

When the patient is old, weak, or poorly motivated, treatment is not advisable. The exercises and effort required are laborious, frequently boring, and must be done often and regularly. Results, even after a great deal of work, can be so limited that the feasibility of undertaking this program needs to be carefully assessed, especially if the fee creates a difficulty for the family. If the dysarthric has a progressive disease such as Muscular Sclerosis or Amyotropic Lateral Sclerosis, speech therapy cannot ward off the steady deterioration of muscle usage in these illnesses. A dysarthric patient will remain dysarthric in spite of the best possible treatment, but significant improvement of intelligibility can be achieved by some people, and this can certainly make life more worthwhile. When a patient is young, strong, and highly motivated, capable of carrying out a rigorous course of training, such a program should be undertaken if the speech pathologist feels his condition can be improved by this action.

Can a Layman Help Him to Speak More Clearly?

Without initial diagnosis and guidance by a speech pathologist it would be difficult for a layman to know what to do to improve intelligibility. A series of exercises must be started, designed to strengthen and improve the use of those muscles needed to produce specific speech sounds more clearly. Each program must be planned for the individual, as there are many variations of muscle weakness and paralysis.

Someone who is with the patient regularly can be trained by the therapist to work with the patient daily and to give him invaluable feedback. During the early weeks of therapy, a patient is often unable to tell when he is doing something correctly or is headed in that direction. Guidance by another person to the proper movements and sounds is important, but that person must know exactly what goals are being pursued. Only "perfect practice makes perfect." Many dysarthric patients practice daily, but incorrectly, and therefore nothing is accomplished. The brain injury causing dysarthria may affect judgment. It may also have damaged other channels through which we get information about how different parts of our bodies are functioning. For example, the patient may have lost some sensation in the areas where the muscles are impaired so he does not fully feel what his face, lips, tongue, throat, and other body parts are doing.

If nasality is present certain activities can be carried out at home that may strengthen the weakened muscles and help produce clearer speech. For example, the muscles needed to close off the nasal passages and prevent nasality are put to use when blowing through the mouth. Therefore, blowing feathers, light bits of paper, bubble pipes, and, much later, balloons, are fine ways of exercising those muscles. However, it is necessary to be certain that the air setting feathers and paper into motion is not being emitted through the nostrils. If it is, the effort will be entirely wasted. Closing off the patient's nostrils with fingers while he is blowing can prevent this. It must be impressed upon him that the seal has to be tight or the exercise is of no value.

When nasality is very severe because many muscles are extremely impaired, it is possible that the patient will not be able to blow air through his mouth with enough force to stir even the lightest of feathers. There are prosthetic devices than can be used in some extreme cases of nasality, and these need to be carefully evaluated by physician and speech pathologist.

Few if any of us use all of our muscles to the utmost of their capability. So also with the dysarthric patient; but if he is to improve at all, the necessity for using his speech muscles as well as his disability allows is critical. Perfection of production need not be the goal, unless it is within his ultimate capability, but rather the best approximation his muscles will allow. That must be his daily target, reaching ever finer adjustments with the regular exercise. And as with all other forms of exercise, the more regularly these muscles are used, the easier the task becomes.

The most important contributions a layman can make are not only to see that the prescribed therapy program is correctly done, but that when the dysarthric has reached a better level of production of a particular group of sounds, he uses those sounds correctly whenever he talks. If this means that he is ignored when he talks in his old mushy, slurred way after he has demonstrated that he can talk more clearly, then that is what must be done. It also means that he should receive rewards of special attention when he talks well.

How Can Ice Be Used to Help Some Forms of Dysarthria?

Physical and occupational therapists use ice on muscles of the body under certain circumstances, to help these muscles perform better. It has been found that when the muscles used for swallowing are so weakened that a patient drools and has difficulty swallowing food, a program of applying ice in particular ways to the muscles of the mouth and face can often produce favorable results. For many of these patients, drooling is eliminated and swallowing food is made easier and safer. Those patients whose speech was very slurred and unintelligible because of the impairment of this particular set of muscles may be helped to speak more clearly, just by the application of ice, and without any additional exercises.

In those progressive diseases such as Amyotropic Lateral Sclerosis (ALS) in which the patient has serious difficulty swallowing, icing will not provide permanent improvement, and it must be very carefully used because the patient may choke on the melting ice. However, I have had reports from families that for as much as a half hour after eating sherbet, some ALS patients' speech became more intelligible, and they were able to use this time for better communication.

Not all physical, occupational, and speech therapists have been trained to apply ice. Not all physicians are knowledgeable of the technique, either. Those who are may automatically order a slush diet for all dysarthric patients. This means that all foods are liquified and mixed with ice in a blender so a solid slush is obtained. The doctors will also order icing of the oral muscles if a therapist is available who has been trained to do it. Icing should only be undertaken with the physician's consent, because the shock of the extreme cold may be dangerous for certain blood pressure and heart conditions. In most cases there is no danger involved, but the decision to carry it out should be a medical one.

It is not yet clear what other forms of dysarthria may be helped by icing. When muscles other than those used for swallowing are involved in a speech impairment, there is no strong evidence that icing is helpful. I automatically order icing for all dysarthric patients whose physicians concur, three times daily if possible, for at least a month. Some seem to improve, others not, and

I have not had an opportunity to conduct a controlled study to determine what other kinds of dysarthria may respond favorably.

Does Dysarthria Ever Improve Long After Onset?

I have known dysarthric patients to improve years after onset when an appropriate course of exercises or icing was introduced that had never been used earlier. Some patients respond better later, even years later, than they do early after onset. They have stabilized and are sometimes stronger physically, so they are better able to carry out an exercise program. Some are better motivated. At the earlier period some patients do not grasp the significance of their injury; they do not understand the permanence of the damage, and, feeling that it will vanish eventually, they are unwilling to expend the effort required to improve their speech. Later they have faced the reality of the impairment and wish very strongly to get help. These conditions are not true of all or even most dysarthrics, but they are not unusual.

Much has been said about the atrophy of muscles when not used for long periods of time, but I am often impressed by patients who have been wheelchair-bound for years, never having consulted a physical therapist, who learn to walk with a cane or walker after a course of physical therapy is introduced. The same improved muscle use can happen to some dysarthrics when treatment is started late.

There are times when patients seem to have recovered as much intelligibility as they are capable of reaching; therefore, terminating treatment appears to be the best course. Some of these patients return several years later, their speech much improved and now seek help to improve even further. In every case something very favorable emotionally had occurred to the patient to make him try harder to speak more clearly. One patient, a man whose wife had divorced him after a stroke and left him wheelchair-bound and dysarthric, had been living in a board and care facility for four years when he returned for further help. I had not seen him for two years and was delighted to find his speech much clearer than when I had last seen him. He had joined a stroke club a year earlier and had met the widow of a former member who had remained actively involved with the club after her husband's death. They were about to get married and his happiness was reflected in his slower, more precise and more intelligible speech.

Chapter XII

Changes Brain Damage Brings to the Family

Are There Certain Changes to Be Anticipated After Brain Damage?

Can the Home Be Made Safe and Functional for the Patient's Use?

When Can the Patient Be Left Home Alone?

When the Husband and Main Breadwinner Suffers the Brain Injury . . . !

When the Housewife Suffers the Brain Injury . . . !

If the Patient Cannot Be Cared for Adequately at Home, What Are the Alternatives?

Does Brain Injury Affect Sexual Feelings? Can Brain Injured People Have Sexual Relations?

What Can Be Done About the Disturbed Feelings of Family Members?

Are There Certain Changes to Be Anticipated After Brain Damage?

For all but the very mildly impaired who soon recover all their former abilities, brain injury necessitates alterations in the lives of the patients and those people closely involved with them. In this final chapter, the most frequently encountered situations are discussed along with some suggested ways of handling them. If families are forewarned that difficulties might arise under certain circumstances, and solutions to these potential problems are planned in advance, they will be more readily available should the need for them materialize. Preparation can help prevent undue tensions; a peaceful, stable environment is the best framework in which the patient can recover communicative ability to his maximum potential. Anxiety and tensions among family members are found to be reflected in the patient's performance, and the best efforts of professional treatment may well be undermined if the emotional climate at home is unsettling. Anticipation can result in prevention.

Can the Home Be Made Safe and Functional for the Patient's Use?

When a family member is about to come home from the hospital, paralyzed or weakened in leg and arm, with reduced ability to communicate, the husband, wife, children, or parents are very often overwhelmed by the multitude of adjustments facing them, not knowing how to go about solving some of the obvious problems, much less finding solutions for all they vaguely anticipate. Problems such as how to cope with a wheelchair in the house, how to handle bathroom use of shower, tub, and toilet, dressing, undressing, even transferring some patients from bed to wheelchair; the daily logistical details that make up a normal household's requirements can loom menacingly for the uninitiated. Those patients who have access to a rehabilitation center soon after onset of brain damage will have the advantage of counseling provided for their families by the physical therapist, occupational therapist, speech pathologist, and any other team member the patient's condition requires. However, the majority of patients probably do not have this advantage and their families may not even be aware that such counseling exists. Therefore they do not know that many ready made solutions are available to them for many of the difficulties they anticipate.

Certain alterations and additions to a house can make enormous differences in providing some independence for the patient and his family. Obviously, the patient who is totally dependent upon a spouse, parent, or grown child for every waking need requires that person to lose his own independence and freedom of activity. By adding a ramp, a handrail, removing scatter rugs or deep shag carpeting, providing special equipment in the shower and at the toilet, lowering a mirror, etc., much can be done toward freeing the patient and his family from some mutual subjections. There are devices that enable a patient with a totally paralyzed arm to cut his own fingernails and his own food, to butter his own bread, and even, in some cases, to put on his own socks and shoes. Velcro fastenings replacing buttons and zippers help many a patient dress without help. There are instruments with which a patient can wash his own toes without help and reach things at a distance above or below, so cans on a high shelf can be brought down or fallen objects can be retrieved without seeking assistance.

The American Heart Association (Appendix A) has an assortment of manuals (Appendix B) that offer solutions to some of the multitude of problems faced by patients with all varieties of physical handicaps. Some solutions are devices and appliances that must be bought, others that can be made. Some are suggestions for rearranging furniture and equipment to improve freedom of movement and safety for the patient. For the patient with paralysis, the manual "Do It Yourself Again; Self-Help Devices For The Stroke Patient" (Appendix B) offers many suggestions along with photographs and drawings that families have found to be especially valuable in guiding them in the reorganization of their household.

The telephone company has some solutions enabling certain patients to use the telephone more easily. A visit to the local office may help the family to solve some of these problems. A fairly new system now available throughout the United States and in some foreign countries can provide peace of mind for many families who must leave the patient home alone, or where the patient is able to live alone. This is an electronic system that makes use of the telephone but is provided by a private company (Microlert Systems, Appendix A). It consists of two parts: part one is plugged into an existing or added phone jack, and part two is worn by the patient at all times. It has no wires so he is free to move wherever he wishes. If he gets into trouble, he needs only to squeeze the pendant he wears and help will be immediately notified. The system will have been programmed to alert whatever person or agency the family desires at the time of installation, a family member, the police, a paramedic team, and so on. The system is not inexpensive, but a consultation with a company representative may provide solutions for certain families, enabling them to purchase this valuable aid. It must be borne in mind that under certain circumstances the system will not be useful. For example, if the patient becomes unconscious, or if he has a sudden stroke on the other side resulting in two handed paralysis, or if under the stress of a catastrophe he forgets about squeezing the pendant, something that brain damaged people may very well do, the system will not be activated.

For the woman who is going to resume some of the household chores again but either needs to do them from her wheelchair or from a seated position for those tasks which require much time, the heights of working surfaces in the kitchen need to be examined. Alterations may be less costly than hiring a servant. Moreover, by enabling her to become useful again, she gains in ability to recover some feelings of self-worth which brain damage often reduces seriously.

One of the important functions of occupational therapy is to retrain patients in activities of daily living. Through the help of occupational therapists (O.T.s) brain injured people can often learn to shave, dress, and to take care of nearly all their personal needs. Learning to control bowel and bladder functions is possible for a great many patients who have not learned to do it because their families did not know these functions can often be retrained. An evaluation by an occupational therapist experienced in dealing with brain injured patients can reveal whether or not a patient has the potential for further recovery of function if he receives some training. It generally takes only a few months of therapy to bring the patient to his optimal level of functioning. The occupational therapist, by making a home visit, can recommend important changes that will provide maximum safety and function for the patient in his daily environment. If there is difficulty locating an O.T., an inquiry can be sent to their national headquarters (see Appendix A).

Physical therapists (P.T.s) help a patient to recover use of the large muscles to whatever extent potential for recovery exists. Patients who might otherwise remain wheelchair-bound are often capable of learning to walk again with the aid of a walker or a cane, if they are evaluated and treated by a physical therapist. Some can learn to walk up and down stairs safely so that new sleeping arrangements do not have to be made at home. Learning to help a patient transfer with safety, alone or with minimal assistance, from bed to wheelchair is a tremendous boon to many families. Too many amateur assistants who have never been properly trained to lift a paralyzed patient, sustain serious and permanent back injuries after months of doing this chore incorrectly daily. Obviously the task need not be injurious if done in the proper way since physical therapists and nurses must do this regularly with many patients, some considerably larger and heavier than themselves. A physical therapist often joins the occupational therapist in making a home visit to suggest ways to improve the home for the patient's use and comfort. The national headquarters of physical therapists (Appendix A) can recommend the nearest available P.T.s.

More than a few patients several years after onset are referred to these therapies or to a speech pathologist, never having been evaluated by any of these professionals earlier. Some can be helped to regain functions that have lain dormant for many months or years. It is sad to realize that a long period of greater freedom and better communicative ability might have been attained by the patient had he received help sooner, but it should be comforting to know that even long after onset, muscles can still be retrained and language ability improved in some people. If no professionals are available in the immediate community, the family should make every effort to learn where they can take the patient for an evaluation by a rehabilitation team. It is worthwhile to pay a visit to a distant center if need be, early after onset if possible; but if this was not done, then it can still be arranged for a previously untreated patient. If the patient was a veteran, he may be entitled to these services at the nearest Veteran's Administration Hospital or outpatient clinic.

When Can the Patient Be Left Home Alone?

One of the traumatic realizations that comes to family members is that their own freedom of movement may be seriously hampered by the new conditions. When a patient is unable to move around without help or to communicate, it is obvious that he cannot be left alone, even for short periods. Some kind of relief must be provided so that the family member is able to go shopping, to go to work if need be, or to have a social engagement away from home. Some families have worked this out by enlisting the help of neighbors, friends, or other relatives when employing assistance is unfeasible. Some fortunate people have developed an arrangement so that no one person needs to be called upon more than once a month, yet there are enough people available volunteering their services so that the spouse, parent, or chlid is relatively free some part of every week to take care of necessary duties.

The patient who can transfer alone from bed to wheelchair or who moves about the house laboriously with cane or walker, and who can use the telephone to summon help, is the one who is often left alone, although certain risks are apparent.

Perhaps the most frequently occurring accident to these mobile but handicapped people is that of falling. Many of them cannot get up without assistance if they fall. Some may actually injure themselves further by striking their heads against hard or pointed surfaces Many family members have described to me their nightmares concerning a relative who lives alone after a stroke: lying helpless following a fall, engulfed in flames in a burning house.

One son I knew called his father several times every day from work due to his sometimes overwhelming anxiety as the fantasy of tragedy striking his parent during the few hours since his last call overcame him. When his father did not answer the phone after a reasonable number of rings, the son would alert neighbors and would sometimes even leave his office to rush to his father's house, often finding that independent gentleman walking leisurely a few blocks from home or visiting with some neighboring children. It was the father who consulted me to find solutions for his son's anxiety so he himself could feel freer to move about the neighborhood. He did not want the indignity of having to call his son every time he left the house, not did he want to cause the young man undue stress, knowing how ultimately injurious to his health it could certainly become. Through counseling, the son finally learned to accept his father's need for independence without submitting himself to stress. One practical solution was to alert neighbors who knew the father well to look in on him if they did not see him out of doors for several hours. The son finally learned to trust the fact that if anything serious happened to his father, one of them would be in touch with him. Fortunately this never had to occur during the long period of time I had contact with this family. Certain risks have to be taken in order to prevent other kinds of damage to self-esteem.

Fire is an ever present danger that must be kept well in mind when deciding the risk of leaving a patient alone, even for a short period. Patients who walk well enough for daily purposes may not have the necessary speed or coordination required in an emergency. Even a patient who appears to be able to talk well enough to use the phone may not be able to do so when he becomes panic-stricken. People who live in elevator buildings should remember that in case of an earthquake or a fire they must never use an elevator. The patient who ambulates with difficulty, or is wheelchair bound, may be trapped in an upper floor unable to use the stairs for escape. It is probably advisable to consider moving to a first floor apartment when there is any ambulation difficulty, if it is at all feasible.

There are times when it is necessary to leave the house on an errand, and preparing a patient to come along may necessitate some burdensome activities. If a friendly neighbor can be alerted that the patient is to be left alone for a specified time, and notified when the person returns, much anxiety and risk can be relieved. It is not always necessary that someone remain in the house with the patient, but it is a good idea for someone nearby to know the patient is alone in case of an emergency; if the period is to be extended for several hours, he should be looked in upon at regular intervals. Some patients can even be left alone all day under these circumstances, especially when the spouse has to work and there is a dependable, willing neighbor to look in frequently—one who knows what to do in case of emergency.

A patient left alone all day—even if his safety has been well provided for—may suffer in other ways, especially in lack of opportunity for communication. An aphasic patient who cannot read or understand speech easily enough to enjoy much television may very well regress in language ability and emotional well-being if left unstimulated daily. Some communities offer day care centers for adults in such situations. There are also closed workshops sponsored by various organizations that offer small paying jobs for handicapped people. These jobs involve tasks such as sorting nails according to size or mending articles donated to charity. The brain injured person who can do this sort of work often gains much in feelings of self-esteem by having a place to go each day where he can do a needed chore and receive pay for it, no matter how small the amount. Some patients who might be able to do these tasks may refuse because the contrast to their former level of performance becomes too painful. I have known patients who refused to go in the early months or even years after onset, but later welcomed the activity, having at long last bowed to the inevitability of their changed status. To locate day care centers or closed workshops, one should inquire of the physician or paramedicals treating the patient, the local chapter of the American Heart Association, the nearest rehabilitation center, or a visiting home health service. If none is offered in a community, there may be enough interest alerted to start such a group, if a sufficient number of people are located who are able to benefit from these services.

Some families with a member who cannot be left alone while others must work or attend school have to pay someone to stay with the patient. For many the pay is exorbitant and unrealistic. In some cases it may be possible to find a student or retired person in the neighborhood who, for a relatively small fee, would consent to be responsible for the patient during certain specified hours. I have known some of these invaluable helpers (who derive much pleasure from taking the patient to his therapy, even receiving the training necessary to help the patient at home) to take the patient to occasions of interest in the community and on outings that provide stimulation and enrichment of the hours that might otherwise be long and dreary.

Sometimes it is easier to find several people, who divide the days into committed times, than to find one person to assume the entire time commitment. By examining one's work demands or class schedule, it is sometimes possible to adjust those duties to arrange for more time spent at home. A wife I knew was able to find a helper for afternoons but none who could attend her husband in the mornings. A conference with her employer provided a fine solution. She was able to perform certain of her duties at home on the telephone just as easily as she could at the office, so arrangements were accordingly made that she work at home until noon daily and then report to the office after the helper appeared.

It is heartening to learn how many people are willing and able to cooperate and provide needed solutions when serious tragedies strike; all that is required at times is to make evident the need for assistance. People who are reluctant to turn to others for help are often the losers. Many individuals feel themselves enriched if they are able to assist in solving problems for overburdened neighbors, acquaintances, or friends. The worst that can happen is that the request for help will be turned down, a minor risk when the alternative result may be problem solution.

When the Husband and Main Breadwinner Suffers the Brain Injury

When the family's income is threatened or cut off because the main provider has been stricken, profound changes are necessarily required. This often means that a wife must suddenly assume responsibilities for which she is poorly prepared. In families oriented toward traditional roles, the husband has not only been the main source of income but has often been the main decision maker. His impairment forces his wife to find ways to keep an income flowing, no matter how curtailed, to deal with problems her background has not prepared her to handle adequately—often without even the knowledge of where to turn for advice, be it legal, economic, or pragmatic in nature. Decisions often have to be made quickly, and at a time when she is under enormous stress emotionally.

In addition to these considerations which she must rapidly learn to manage, there are personal role changes, "balance of power" alterations within the family unit that she must face. Some of these can cause added stress not only for herself in assuming the new responsibilities, but for the patient who feels himself losing status under the altered conditions. A severely impaired patient will not be aware of the necessary shifts, but the mildly or moderately injured patient can be deeply disturbed when he learns of decisions that have been made without his concurrence. Some had to be made while he was still too ill to be consulted, others because his wife, overburdened as she is, has not thought it necessary to consult him, and in her agitation may sell the house or car or other property, select or relinquish an investment, or take some other long range action without discussing it with him. The effect upon her husband can be catastrophic, not only because of the actual decision made but because of his feeling of being pushed out of the control center of his family.

A wife I knew decided that her husband's expensive foreign car was a luxury they could no longer afford. It was obvious that he would never be able to handle it again, and she certainly had no intention of driving it; so she sold it at a very good price, the money received making it possible to provide her husband with the therapies he required. His reaction was so strong that for a time everyone feared he would suffer another stroke or a heart attack. He refused to leave his bed, refused the treatment the money made possible, and his desperate wife came perilously close to a nervous breakdown. Through counseling she realized that the car represented to him the last vestiges of his feelings of power, of his actual masculinity, and by selling it, especially without consulting him, she was, according to his interpretation, telling him that he was now powerless and impotent. Yet she knew realistically that without selling it there was little chance that he would receive the treatment he needed to learn to walk and to communicate better. When she understood what he was coping with emotionally, she found ways to handle the situation well. She did everything possible to defer to him when critical issues were not at stake. She made every attempt to show him how important he was to her and how much she wanted him to get better so he could take over the reins again. In time he accepted the new situation and felt better about himself, able to accept her as a partner and no longer needing to be the sole arbiter.

Very often, under the stresses of the unaccustomed role and kinds of decisions facing her, a wife may forget to give much emotional attention to her husband. As a result, his responses to her actions may be intensified because of his fear of being thrust aside. It is, indeed, difficult to give emotional comfort to someone else when one is filled with one's own fears and anxieties; yet the wife who finds ways to keep her husband from feeling left out, no matter how exhausted she might be from all the new pressures, will usually have an easier time of it at home. By taking time to create a climate in which her husband can maintain self-esteem regardless of how much realistic control he has had to relinquish, a wife will gain much in preserving meaningful qualities of their relationship.

Much of what happens after brain damage strikes depends upon the relationship between the two before the onset of the impairment. When mutual love, trust, respect, and good communication existed earlier, the transition to the shift in roles will be easier in many ways than in those marriages that had problems. A wife who is sensitive to her husband's feelings of loss will want to help him recover and maintain feelings of self worth in every way possible without jeopardizing the well-being of the family. She will make a concerted attempt to keep her husband informed of what she is trying to do, to explain to him the various choices and to give him a part in the decision making, perhaps gently steering him to a wiser choice when his was obviously poorer. He may not understand her words well—perhaps not at all—but he has a good chance of understanding the respect and the desire to share that lie behind the words, and respond favorably to that.

I have known some wives who so fear upsetting their husbands' position as "head of the house" that they become blind to the obvious fact that little or nothing of what they say to their husbands is being understood. A wife whose husband nodded and smiled at everything said to him, after it was clearly demonstrated to her that he had poor understanding, persisted in asking his advice on every step she took. She followed the advice of his seemingly affirmative responses to all of her questions. Until her son took over, she was well on the way to destroying the finances of the family. This was not a basically stupid woman, but rather a woman so conditioned to the role of deferring to her husband that she repressed her knowledge of his inability to comprehend anything that was said to him.

Another woman I knew became the victim of a terrible automobile accident because she refused to take away her husband's driving privileges, although it was obvious that his slow reflexes provided a serious risk if he needed to act quickly while behind the wheel. His driver's license was not yet up for renewal, so she was able to permit him to drive with the rationalization that he still had bona fida permission from the state to do this. One day he was unable to apply the brakes in time to prevent a catastrophe. She did not survive, but he did, and is now in a nursing home, much more seriously brain damaged, and quite alone.

Through the years I have known some husbands who seemed almost content in their impairment. I am not necessarily referring to a state of euphoria but rather to a willing and even seemingly happy acceptance of dependency and freedom from decision making, much to the amazement and chagrin of those who knew them in their pre-impairment days. Who can say what former stresses they had been under that make brain damage a condition that brings them peace at last? Of course, brain injury itself often prevents people from perceiving reality. It can distort time. Many of these patients may not be aware of the seriousness or permanence of their condition.

The majority of patients I have treated have responded reasonably well to their new status. They relinquish family control as needed, they work hard to improve in all possible functions, and they are very cooperative in the hospital and after they go home, not making unreasonable demands upon their wives, but attempting in every way possible to lighten the burden. I have tried to present here the most frequent problems that can arise. Some aspects of these may appear periodically in the responses of very reasonable patients.

In some cases of brain injury, the patient may be trained to handle another type of job when he cannot return to the kind of work he was doing. If this appears to be possible, consultation with a vocational rehabilitation counselor is a wise course to pursue. If none is available in the immediate community the National Rehabilitation Association (Appendix A) can provide information for locating this service.

When the Housewife Suffers the Brain Injury

Whatever was the realm of responsibility of the brain-injured person, that domain must suffer the loss of that person's services, either temporarily or permanently. When the housewife and mother loses her ability to communicate, to move around as before, to run the household with its multitude of varied chores and the skills this necessitates—when she can no longer be the cook, housekeeper, laundress, hostess, marketer, and taxi service she once was, someone or several must assume these roles. Often the husband must do it all, or try to, along with his own responsibilities. The burden becomes great.

The brain injured wife, as the brain injured husband, often feels a great loss of personal worth that will have its affect upon her personality. Most will be eager to please and will cooperate well. Some will become withdrawn and depressed, while others will be angry and unreasonable. Many will take turns with all these reactions. In our society there is great emphasis upon a woman's physical appeal; therefore, often more so than among men, a woman is apt to feel a strong loss of body image when she suffers paralysis or weakness of parts of her body. She may lose the feeling that her husband can find her attractive and desirable, and this can certainly influence her behavior.

The problems these conditions create for the overburdened husband can be enormous. At a time when he is learning to cope with all the additional responsibilities, even more so if there are small children involved, he must also see to it that his wife feels he still finds her attractive. Nothing may be further from his mind than being an ardent lover, not because of his reaction to her condition necessarily, but because of the emotional and physical strains of his daily life; yet unless he gives her physical proof that she is still desirable to him, he may find himself with an additional domestic crisis on his hands. If a husband will take a few minutes to go out of his way to touch his wife lovingly, to smile and wink at her, to drop a kiss on her head or cheek while he is rushing to bathe the children or perform some other domestic duty after his long day at the office, this small attention may do much to make life more peaceful at home.

Humor and keeping things in perspective can work wonders to prevent tensions from building and to create a climate in which the patient as well as other family members may perform in an easy relaxed way. If the husband arrives home tense and driven from his working day and hurries to get the evening chores out of the way so he can relax, he will be apt to multiply greatly the difficulties and tensions of the household. If he takes time to visit with his wife and children, perhaps having a leisurely drink, delaying dinner, and giving them all a chance to enjoy one another, he can help to create a pleasant, loving home environment in which his wife and children can thrive. Food may not be gourmet, baths may have to be skipped, but the climate created will encourage everyone to perform better, and that will pay big dividends. Children given responsibilities along with love and humor can perform amazingly responsible tasks.

There can be negative reactions among children. They may repress resentment they feel toward their disabled mother because she is no longer available to them as before, but sometimes their hostility is thinly veiled. If the father understands this and can discuss it openly and honestly with them, much can be done to alleviate the feelings as well as the troubles these feelings produce.

When a wife's former responsibilities can be given to others by hiring people to take over these chores, it can greatly simplify the logistics of the situation. Not all families are in a position to assume such expensive solutions. Often other family members must be called upon to assist. Neighbors and friends may be enlisted to help in providing transportation to therapies, to physicians, and to drill the patient at home in language assignments. There are many people who would like nothing better than to provide some form of help, but they do not know what or even if they should offer. One person can be placed in charge of finding recruits and assigning to them their responsibilities. If enough people can be found, no one need be called upon very often—perhaps only once a month for a few hours.

A fine group of solutions to many problems is well presented in the book *Pat and Roald* (Farrell, 1969), the account of the actress Patricia Neal, her writer husband, Roald Dahl, and their children, from the time of her stroke when she was three months pregnant. The book sensitively follows the family through the birth of her fourth child and for several years thereafter until she was finally able to return to her career. The emotional fluctuations and interactions of the entire family are keenly depicted, as well as the methods designed by Roald to involve others in regular assignments to work with his wife on different aspects of her language and memory problems. The rich social interactions are given prominence also, as they played an important role in keeping her in touch with good communication situations. Other books of this nature can also be found in the local libraries, written by families of brain injured patients, and even by the recovered patients themselves (Wulf, 1973). They generally provide interesting reading and give a perspective not easily found elsewhere to a troubled family.

Because brain damage can interfere with good judgment, some patients may attempt to do things that result in tragedy. The home is statistically the scene of most accidents, and there are many opportunities for the brain injured housewife to perform tasks that have unhappy endings. The aphasic, hemiparetic mother of three young children, all under age seven, one day tried to carry a pot of newly brewed coffee from the stove to the table in her left hand, since her right hand was weak. She limped, and her husband was adamant that she never try to carry any cooked food to the table from the stove, but to wait instead until he came to carry the served food to each place. On this particular morning she unwisely decided to surprise him by having everything ready for him when he came to breakfast. As she neared the table, she tripped and lost control of the coffee pot. All three of the little faces around the table were scalded by the boiling hot coffee splashing over them, as were her arm and legs.

Is there a way to avoid such tragedies? Hindsight offers solutions. Perhaps if she had been made to feel more accepted and worthwhile, she might not have needed to prove her capability by choosing such an unwise method for demonstration. Her husband later admitted that he felt so overburdened and exhausted that he often had little patience with her, speaking to her shortly, even critically many times, for things she could not possibly help. He realized at last her frantic need to prove herself, to take over more responsibilities, hoping therefore to lighten his burden.

When dealing with human beings there are two sets of issues to identify: the practical ones and the emotional ones. The latter are far more difficult to identify and solve. A brain injured person remains subject to all the emotional ramifications that loss of former functions and status imposes on anyone. When the significant persons in the life of that patient care enough to try to understand what she is feeling and attempting to cope with, many good solutions can emerge. When this sensitivity is lacking, problems not only remain but generally multiply.

If the Patient Cannot Be Cared for Adequately at Home, What Are the Alternatives?

Nursing homes or board and care facilities are solutions, of course. They must be carefully investigated to be sure they provide a clean, sanitary, comfortable environment, with satisfactory food, and a caring, well-trained staff who know how to handle brain damaged patients. Good facilities, however, are not inexpensive, which presents another very realistic problem.

Many husbands or wives insist on keeping their mates at home even when it is obviously becoming too difficult to care for them adequately. I have known many a husband or wife, crippled with arthritis or with slipped discs in their spinal column causing them excruciating pain, with palsied hands, or with their own health threatened by heart attack or stroke, trying with superhuman effort to continue caring for their wheelchair-bound mate, so that neither of them is getting proper care.

For some who insist on maintaining this unrealistic arrangement, the alternative of facing the empty, useless days ahead without someone to care for is more than he or she can contemplate. For others, the guilt feelings they experience at the thought of such a solution are too painful to permit them to take this step. Some are carrying out a promise made to their mates at a better time never to put them into such places, so at all costs now they wish to fulfill this promise.

Tragically some of these patients outlive their worn out mates by years, and have had to be placed into homes among strangers with no caring person checking the conditions. If the spouse had selected the place earlier, a more suitable environment might have been located and the patient could have become accustomed to it and the other patients while still receiving frequent visits from his mate.

When caring for a handicapped relative produces disabilities or increases existing ones, the time to consider alternative solutions has arrived, while the choice can still be made. Some people cannot make the choice because they fear anger, rejection, and criticism from other relatives. Someone who has been ruled all of his life by fear of the opinions of others may have particularly hard times. Only if he can be made fully aware that it is in the patient's best interest to be placed into a home and that others agree, can he make the final decision.

Most patients who find themselves in a good nursing home finally adjust satisfactorily. The comfort and care they experience are so superior to what they were getting at home that they generally finally accept it, even gratefully, especially if the family remains unmoved by early entreaties to rescue them. Many even learn to enjoy it because of the greater stimulation they find there compared to the lonely, isolated situation at home with only their exhausted mate for company.

People who live alone and—obviously to their loved ones—can no longer be considered safe to continue this arrangement after suffering brain injury, may present their own resistance against a change. Those who are ambulatory and have long been used to independence often fight vigorously to maintain their accustomed household. When it becomes clear to others that they are not eating proper meals (malnutrition is common among the elderly or disabled who live alone) or are in constant danger of falling, of forgetting to light the gas they have turned on, of letting things burn in pots on the stove because they have forgotten it was cooking, or any of the other risks threatening brain injured people, steps must be taken to convince them a change is necessary.

For some, a paid companion may provide a fine solution, and perhaps be even less expensive than a board and care facility. Unfortunately, someone who has long lived alone does not always accept a stranger into her household graciously. She may be unable to prepare a satisfactory meal herself, but resent the presence of this unwelcomed person in her kitchen. I am reminded of a delightful but stubborn elderly patient I had who went through 15 paid companions in short order, finding imaginary fault with each of them, until one day she herself succeeded in providing the solution. The day after firing the fifteenth companion she prepared a simple stew for herself and then left the house to take a walk in the nearby park. The day was lovely and she enjoyed watching children at play, so she forgot the meal she had left cooking on the stove. When she returned home sometime later, much of the house had been destroyed by fire. The board and care home the family found for her allowed her complete freedom to come and go as she liked, but provided all her meals, laundry service, household chores, and available medical care if needed. When she found that no one offered sympathy for her string of complaints, she at last permitted herself to make friends there among the other boarders, and admitted to me that she was actually enjoying herself, after I promised not to confess this to her family.

Does Brain Injury Affect Sexual Feelings? Can Brain Injured People Have Sexual Relations?

When there is no paralysis, weakness, or loss of sensation in any part of the body following onset, there need be no change in any sexual response experienced by a brain injured person. If changes are encountered, they are likely to be due either to psychological factors or to the effects of some medications. The latter may be solved by asking the physician if there is an alternative medication that may not interfere with sexual responses. Psychological factors are more complex.

Even with paralysis and loss of sensation, sexual feelings and responses need not always suffer much change. Human sexual response has strong survival capability, so even with muscular and sensory losses in some parts of the body, there are generally enough remaining areas capable of responding that satisfactory sexual experiences are still possible for most people. Adjustments to the new limitations have to be made, but when there is adequate understanding of what is required, most people can make the necessary changes to their mutual satisfaction.

The first question uppermost in the minds of each patient and sexual partner, too often not put to the physician because of shyness and reluctance to discuss this area of intimacy, is whether or not sexual activity will be safe. If there were any need to curtail sexual activity, the physician would have made that abundantly clear before the patient left the hospital. As a general rule, there is no danger whatsoever, so many physicians do not even mention sex unless it is necessary to place limitations upon it, or unless the patient or the patient's mate asks. A frank discussion with the physician is sensible if there are questions.

Because of the paralysis (unilateral if due to stroke, often bilateral if due to other causes), positioning of the body becomes a major consideration in the new conditions. Couples who had good sexual communication before the onset of brain injury soon find ways in which both can comfortably enjoy sexual contact with one another, accommodating to the new conditions as necessary. Those who always had problems revealing to each other their sexual preferences will have greater difficulties now. It is a pity that people are often reluctant to admit to discomfort, pain, or preference for a different position in sexual situations, when they would not hesitate to express it in some other circumstance.

Some sexual partners too easily take offense and believe themselves to be rejected when the partner expresses discomfort. There are couples who have had no sexual relations for many years following the advent of brain injury, because early experiences were so uncomfortable for the patient that the "healthy" partner never dared to approach him or her again. If, instead, both had tried honestly and openly to find ways of experiencing pleasure in greater comfort, many years of important sexual release and communication could have been theirs. If the patient has a language problem severe enough to prevent verbal communication, there are many nonverbal ways of notifying the partner of pleasing and non-pleasing acts. A partner sensitive to these cues will make adjustments as often as necessary until the best arrangement can be found. Many people are conditioned to sexual responses in one position only. The need to find new positions in which to have sexual relations may, for them, be utterly out of the question emotionally. It is unfortunate for both parties, since they are the losers in this rigid psychological attitude, but without psychiatric or counseling intervention, not much can be done to solve their problem.

When the male has suffered paralysis, the woman generally has to become more aggressive in the sexual act. For some women this is a very difficult role to assume. Some male patients who have been especially strongly conditioned to the male supremacy role in sexual union find it humiliating for their wives to become aggressive sexually, and this reaction may lead to impotency, even if handled with great sensitivity. This problem may need psychiatric treatment, which can be difficult for someone with limited communicative ability.

Paralysis sometimes produces spasms, contractions, and heightened reflexes in the paralyzed areas. If these occur during the sexual act, both partners may be frightened enough never to try again, not understanding that this is a possible, but not serious consequence of the paralysis. The event may produce too much pain for continuation of the act at that time, but it should certainly not prohibit future contact. Frequent experiences of contractions and spasms, whether or not accompanying the sexual act, should be brought to the physician's attention. There are sometimes steps he can take medically to reduce or eliminate their occurrence.

Incontinence of bowel and bladder, especially in women, is a frequent accompaniment to paralysis or muscle weakness. Psychological reaction to this may interfere with sexual response. However, if both partners are aware of the possibility and make certain that bowel and bladder are emptied before sexual acts begin, there is lessened likelihood of any embarrassment during intercourse. If it should occur, the partner who can remain calm, loving, and reassuring to the mate can accomplish a great deal in preventing future sexual withdrawal; otherwise the brain injured person may become so fearful of this occurrence that sex will be strongly avoided from then on. Of course, if the uninjured partner is repelled enough by the possibility, no sexual response to the mate may be forthcoming in the future—an unfortunate consequence of negative conditioning to natural acts in our society.

Some men may experience impotence after the onset of brain damage. If stroke is the cause of the injury, hemiplegia alone should not cause impotence; however, when thrombosis produced the stroke, a clogging of the arteries leading to the sexual organs may be suspected as a cause. The impotence might have been evident before the stroke occurred, and if it had been reported to a physician at that time, steps might have been taken to relieve it as well as to prevent the stroke; but many men are reluctant to confess this state to their physician, another unfortunate consequence of our conditioning. Since some medications may produce impotence, this possibility should be discussed with the physician. Psychological factors are often the main cause of impotence after a stroke. In other causes of brain injury impotence is sometimes the result of widespread loss of sensation and paralysis.

Brain injury sometimes produces a lack of control over sexual response, an indifference to the sexual needs or responses of the partner that can cause serious disruption of marital relationships. Severe brain damage can alter the character and personality of the patient to such an extent that it might even be dangerous to continue to live with him. For several years after an accident that produces brain damage, a patient can continue to improve so much that he or she may return to former personality status; but during the early years it may not be advisable to attempt to have any kind of a relationship with certain patients, especially a sexual one.

Wives of some stroke patients complain that their husbands have become "selfish" since the stroke, not caring about their (the wives') feelings and wanting to have sex often through the day and even frequently through the night. These may be men who do not reach orgasm, but have a frequently recurring desire for intercourse, unable to find relief through the act. If their wives would relieve them manually or orally, they might be content for days thereafter, but too often the wives are unable to use these sexual techniques due to early conditioning against them, so that they both suffer needlessly. If, however, wives try everything they can think of and cannot bring their husbands to orgasm, the physician should be told. There may be medical reasons for this condition that he can relieve.

Premature ejaculation is another possible result of brain injury, even among men who were well able to insure their wives' sexual satisfaction before the injury. Again the physician should be notified because there may be a medical problem causing it. If it is due to the patient's lack of ability to react to his wife with sensitivity because of the brain injury, she may be able to find ways to help him alter his behavior if she understands what is causing the problem. If his behavior in other situations is sensitive and appropriate, as it was before the onset, and the lack of control is only evident in the sexual situation, there are certain techniques that may be tried to help him regain his former behavior. Seeking guidance of a sexuality counselor may produce happy results. If, however, insensitivity and lack of control is evident in most of his other responses, not much can be done to change the situation, unless time and healing bring it about.

The brain injured wife is usually more concerned at first with her husband's love and acceptance of her new physical disabilities than she is with her own sexual responses. Her first night at home after onset of the disability is often a critical night in setting the tone for the remainder of the couple's sexual relationship, in much the same way that the honeymoon often is. What happens very often if the husband has not been adequately counseled is a scenario much like the following:

The husband brings his newly disabled wife home from the hospital with great trepidations about his ability to cook, to keep the house in order, to take proper physical care of her, to provide for the children's emotional and physical needs if they are young, and to allow himself needed emotional space for his own very urgent needs, such as time to think, to read, to laugh, to meet with his male friends, and all the other small but important events in the course of an average week. By the time he has managed to circumvent all of his fantasized pitfalls of that first day successfully, and has managed to tuck her safely into bed (perhaps the children too have had to be deposited into their rooms for the night), he might be inclined to relax alone in a darkened living room, letting the tensions release themselves before he tries to sleep. His wife, however, has been tensely awaiting his reaction to her as a bed partner. She has decided that his rejection or acceptance of her at that time will confirm or deny her worst fears. His apparent reluctance to join her in bed may bring her to the unfortunate and not necessarily accurate conclusion that he finds her new condition repulsive, that he rejects her as a woman. Her emotional reaction then may be catastrophic, much to his horror. He may be totally unable to understand why she has become hysterical, just when he believed everything had gone quite well.

Adequate counseling before he took her home might have prepared him so that he would have done things very differently. For example, he might have made certain that everything possible would have been taken care of long ahead of time so that he had little to do that first day that would make extra demands upon his own emotional and physical energies. Perhaps after greeting their mother and welcoming her home, the children might have been sent to a relative's house for the first night. He might have arranged for a special meal he had only to reheat, for flowers, for a particular token of his love with a small gift waiting for her on the pillow, and most important of all, joined her in bed soon after she entered it for the night. Whether or not sexual union actually took place that night was not so important to her peace of mind as his holding her and demonstrating that he did not find her unacceptable physically. Even if aphasia prevented her from comprehending the words he said, she could well understand the feeling tone behind the words and react favorably to them.

People suffering from brain injury can become parents. Brain injury itself does not make reproduction impossible. Therefore, unless a child is desired, sexual responsibility must be maintained to assure that a pregnancy does not result if not wanted. The brain injured person often is unable to assume this level of responsibility; therefore, it becomes entirely the duty of the "healthy" partner to make the decision and take the necessary steps to prevent a pregnancy.

A brain injured wife I knew became pregnant although she had been given birth control pills and had been carefully drilled by her physician in the correct use of them, as had her husband. Warned that her memory was not dependable, her husband assumed the responsibility of giving her a pill each morning according to schedule, so he felt secure that a pregnancy—which the doctor warned might be fatal to her—would not occur. None of us was sufficiently tuned in to her state of mind to realize that she felt another child might be just what was needed to keep their marriage together, because she had been having feelings that her husband was beginning to find her undesirable. Because of the brain damage, her reasoning was not completely logical. She knew that a pregnancy was dangerous for her. Moreover, she could not anticipate all the added difficulties another child might present to their family situation. She had managed to keep from swallowing the daily pill until she could dispose of it away from her husband's vigilance, and therefore was able to become pregnant in spite of her husband's responsible preventative measures.

Before a brain injured woman is permitted to become pregnant, her physician should be consulted to determine the risk to her life a pregnancy might present. In certain cases, such as hypertension, the risk may be too great to allow a pregnancy to occur. The woman, herself, should certainly be positive that she wants to undertake this endeavor, and the man must realize that a great deal of the burden in the months ahead will fall upon him. Pregnancy can produce difficulties for both even in the best of circumstances, but a woman who has some paralysis or whose memory, reflexes, and communication ability are impaired will most certainly present problems that will involve him. Moreover, her ability to care for an infant must be minutely considered, unless there is ample financial ability to provide nursing assistance. The wife of a brain damaged man who wants to have a child needs to consider the family unit's ability to provide for the child financially during the period she is unable to work. She must carefully assess the possible effect upon that child of an impaired father, but often these situations work out well. When everything is considered in advance and both decide that a child is wanted and can be cared for adequately, a loving home is more important for the well being of a child than a physically intact brain.

The sexual response of the uninjured partner cannot be dismissed here. Sometimes the spouse, male or female, cannot respond to the patient sexually because of a very real aversion to the distorted body. These are not necessarily unusual reactions, especially in a society which places a high premium on physical beauty and sexual attractiveness. The person who finds himself or herself responding this way to a mate may be overcome with feelings of self-loathing, of guilt, depression, and hopelessness. This person is greatly in need of counseling, which may be able to help him overcome the aversion or accept it and take necessary steps to deal with it. In some cases just knowing oneself not to be a heartless monster, but to realize the reactions are not unusual, alleviates enough guilt for more positive reactions to begin to emerge.

There are marriages that perhaps should be dissolved after brain damage strikes one of the mates. In addition to the obvious changes certain forms of brain damage can produce which make it dangerous to continue living with the patient, there are other changes that make a marriage relationship meaningless. When a patient is severely aphasic so that there is no future possibility of any communication taking place at any level, the "healthy" mate's needs should be considered. After years of a long, good marriage, when misfortune strikes one of the partners the other is not likely to forsake him because of his total disability. However, a marriage that had serious problems developing before the onset of brain injury is generally going to be further disrupted after the disability strikes. A mate who feels trapped is not likely to provide the possible care for the disabled patient. Sometimes a clean break is the best solution for both, rather than subjecting each to years of silent agony.

What Can Be Done About the Disturbed Feelings of Family Members?

Profound changes necessarily take place in the lives of the families of brain injured people. Husbands and wives are hard hit, but so are parents and children, small or grown. All suffer keenly. After the initial shock is past, the new responsibilities are assumed and handled in more or less satisfactory ways. Only then does the reality of permanent change begin to emerge. This change cannot be minimized. Almost no segment of daily living can remain untouched by the event.

Whoever assumes responsibility for the patient may face many hours of fear, isolation, loneliness, fatigue, nervousness, sleeplessness . . . then anger, frustration, and guilt. Resentment toward the patient for becoming ill catches many people by surprise, but it is a frequent reaction. They become greatly distressed that they could have such an appalling response; they may be ashamed to admit it, and, overpowered by guilt, feel themselves to be monsters.

It helps some people to learn that this resentment toward the patient is human and normal. Since it is not unusual to experience a strong anger toward a loved one who dies, why should it not occur toward one who lives, but in such an altered state as to become an entirely different person very often, altogether changing the life-style and future plans of the uninjured relative. Emotional reactions are not legislated. Anger and resentment are the honest and universal effects of unwanted, unplanned, unwelcomed changes. How these feelings are handled, however, can very well affect the lives of all concerned.

The most important first step is to recognize the true nature of the feelings; not to deny them, not to bury them or pretend they do not exist. Buried resentment and anger are apt to emerge in disguised form, or to be directed toward the wrong person or things, very often toward oneself. Psychologists have found that many suicides are the result of repressed anger toward another person, so buried as to be unrecognized as anger, but appearing in the form of deep depression. This anger, redirected toward oneself, may result in self-loathing and hopelessness.

Family members may become martyrs to the patient, doing many things for him that he might otherwise have learned to do for himself. Martyrdom is usually the result of strongly repressed negative feelings toward the patient giving rise to guilt feelings which also go unrecognized. When many daily chores are done for the patient by the martyred relative, that relative feels good; he experiences a relaxation, actually of his guilt feelings, of which he is not really aware. But then he must do something more for the patient and more resentment results. It becomes a vicious circle. The more that is done for the patient, the more dependent the patient becomes, necessitating more tasks being done for him; the one who does these alternates between negative feelings at being a virtual slave to the tasks, guilt feelings at this response, and feelings of relaxation after doing the tasks because the guilt feelings are soothed by the actions. More and more must be done to alleviate some of the bad feelings that continue to arise.

A patient who was three years post onset was brought to me by his wife for the first evaluation of his language disorder he had ever received. She was facing surgery on her spine and needed to find a place for him to stay until she could care for him again, so he was accepted in the nursing home care ward of the hospital on whose staff I was employed. He was eneuretic, incontinent of bowels, wheelchair bound, and could not feed, shave, or dress himself. He did not appear to understand much that was said and did not communicate much verbally. He could be described as demented in many of his actions as he often put everything into his mouth while laughing inappropriately. He had never had any kind of rehabilitative therapy.

His test results indicated that he should be able to communicate at a much higher level that he was presently doing, so a trial period of speech therapy was begun. He was evaluated by occupational and physical therapists who also found that he had potential for a higher level of performance, and they began treatment also. In a matter of a few months his bowel and bladder training were completed and he was no longer incontinent. Soon after this he was walking with the help of a walker and later with only a cane. He learned to shave, bathe, dress, and feed himself. Quite dramatically, he began to comprehend well things that were said to him. All signs of dementia disappeared. His speech was very apraxic as well as aphasic, but after a while he learned to say a few meaningful words. He began to read many words so he could point to them in his notebook when he could not say them.

I spent many hours counseling his wife during her convelescence. She finally faced her strong guilt feelings over the deep resentment she felt toward him for "trapping her" with his brain injury. She realized that only by becoming his slave, although enslaving him also in the process, could she soothe some of these unrecognized but strong negative reactions. She also realized that she was in a sense revenging herself upon him by making him into a useless, demented being. Then she finally became aware of how destructive her actions had been, not only toward him, but to herself. After several years of handling a large, uncooperative man without learning the correct ways of lifting and transferring him from bed to chair, her back was so badly injured that surgery was the only solution.

The revelations were devastating to her at first, but soon she felt great relief. She was more than ready to give up the martyr's role, especially when she saw how independent he could become. At last she was looking forward to having him come home to the new life they could share when she fully recovered.

A brain injured person cannot be confronted with a relative's anger about his condition, but that relative needs to discuss these feelings with someone who understands the problem, preferably a professional counselor. Friends or relatives may be empathetic but there is danger of personal bias toward such confessions, no matter how loving and concerned that friend might be.

Not all marriages were happy ones before the brain damage occurred. Not all children, small or grown, were devoted to the injured parent before the onset, nor was every parent happy in the parenting role before their son or daughter became impaired. People who were unhappy in a relationship before the damage took place will not feel any more kindly toward the patient when they consider themselves to be trapped by the new circumstances. Some couples were actually on the verge of a divorce when the brain injury struck. The big question then is whether to go ahead with the plans, risking incurring everyone's scorn, or to put aside one's own chance for a satisfying life by remaining with the patient. People with these conflicts do well if they seek professional help to try to arrive at a comfortable solution.

Those people who had good, loving relationships with the patient before the tragedy occurred will not be apt to lose that love, but will try in all the possible positive ways to be of help, including assisting the patient to regain the independence of which he is capable. However, even these people will sometimes be aware of some very negative feelings toward the patient, loving him while hating the burden his condition has imposed upon their lives, and sometimes disliking him too. Nearly everyone can recall disliking a beloved parent or friend at one time or another; so it is entirely possible to love the patient deeply while hating his condition and even him at times. By recognizing and accepting the feelings, they can be dealt with and will not arise in unrecognized forms to produce tensions and unaccountable behavior.

Appendix A

Agencies

American Heart Association. 7320 Greenville Avenue, Dallas, Texas, 75231.

American Occupational Therapy Association. 6000 Executive Boulevard, Suite 200, Rockville, Maryland, 20852.

American Physical Therapy Association. 1156 15th Street, NW, Washington, D.C., 20005.

American Speech and Hearing Association. 10801 Rockville Pike, Rockville, Maryland, 20852.

Microlert Systems International. 3030 Empire Avenue, Burbank, California, 91504.

National Rehabilitation Association. 1522 K Street, NW, Washington, D.C., 20005.

Appendix B

Manuals

These may be obtained from the American Heart Association. Single copies are available free.

Aphasia and the Family. Publication #50002A
Do It Yourself Again; Self Help Devices for the Stroke Patient. Publication #50005A.
Strike Back at Stroke. Publication #50024A.
Strokes: Why Do They Behave That Way? Publication #50035A.
Up and Around Again. Publication #50026A.

Glossary of Terms

ADL (pronounced as separate letters). *Activities of Daily Living* such as dressing, shaving, combing one's hair, and bathing. Occupational therapists often need to retrain certain patients in these basic functions.

APHASIA. Partial or total loss of ability to communicate with others through the use of language. Aphasic impairment includes expression by means of speech, writing, and gestures, or reception of the thoughts of others through their spoken, written, or gestural language. Calculation and telling time may also be impaired.

APRAXIA. Loss of ability to carry out purposeful, voluntary movements without the presence of paralysis, muscular weakness, or an impairment of sensation.

1. *apraxia of speech*. Loss of voluntary ability to place the muscles that are needed to produce speech (lips, tongue, mouth, etc.) in correct positions and sequence in order to form words correctly. Placement of these same muscles is correct when used for other purposes, such as eating.

2. *constructional apraxia*. Inability to copy simple drawings or to reproduce patterns created by others with such things as colored blocks.

3. *oral apraxia*. Loss of ability to move the muscles of the mouth correctly when attempting deliberately to stick out the tongue, round or retract the lips, blow, etc., although these same actions can be done easily when used for other purposes.

4. *motor apraxia*. Inability to use an object properly although the nature and purpose of the object is recognized.

5. *sensory apraxia* (also called ideational apraxia). Inability to use an object properly because the nature and purpose of the object is not recognized.

CEREBRUM (CEREBRAL). The largest portion of the brain, divided into two hemispheres, left and right, each of which controls the muscles and integrates sensations on the opposite side of the body. Cognitive, intellectual, and creative functioning take place here, with each

hemisphere taking primary responsibility for certain types of functions.
1. *dominant hemisphere*. The left hemisphere in right-handed people
and the right for left-handed people. Most people have their language
centers in the left hemisphere regardless of dominance.

CVA (pronounced as separate letters). Cerebral vascular accident or
stroke. These terms mean the same thing: that an accident has occurred
in an artery cutting off blood supply to the brain cells fed by that artery
and, therefore, cutting off the function controlled by those particular
brain cells. The accident can be due to a clot, to a narrowing of the
channel caused by thickening of the walls, to a hemorrhage of the artery,
or to a spasm.

DEMENTIA. Impairment of many or all higher brain functions; mental
deterioration with impaired orientation to people, place, and time, along
with impaired memory and judgment. Decrease in one or two of these
abilities does not imply dementia is present.

DIAGNOSIS. Determination of the nature of a disease or other impairment by a professional with specific training to make this determination.

DYSARTHRIA. A disorder of speech and voice production due to
damage to the brain cells controlling the muscles needed to produce
speech and voice, leaving those muscles weak or paralyzed.

EDEMA. Collection of fluid in tissues of the body. When this occurs in
the brain following a stroke or other insult to brain tissue, the
accumulation of fluid can interfere to a varying degree with brain cell
functioning.

EMBOLISM. A clot or plug of any material carried through the blood
vessels to a narrowed section where it suddenly lodges and obstructs
further movement of the bloodstream.

EUPHORIA. Used here as a term describing a condition found in some
some brain injured people who display abnormal, unfounded feelings of
well-being, contentment, and pleasure in the presence of an obvious
serious handicap.

HEMIPARESIS. Impairment of control of the limbs on one side of the
body due to damage to the brain cells controlling voluntary movement of
the involved muscles.

HEMIPLEGIA. Paralysis of limbs on one side of the body due to damage
to the brain cells controlling voluntary movement of the muscles on that
side.

LABILITY (LABILE). A form of emotional instability in which the
patient laughs or cries, often without control, in what appear to be
inappropriate situations. Some brain injured people display this
behavior.

LANGUAGE. Any means we use with which to communicate with others,
especially speech, understanding of speech, reading, writing, and
gestures.

PARAPLEGIC. Paralysis of the lower half of the body on both sides, usually associated with spinal cord injury.

PERSEVERATION. Repetition of a behavior when it is no longer the correct or appropriate response, such as repeating the same word in answer to a series of different questions.

PROGNOSIS. A forecast of the probable course and ultimate termination of a disease or impairment made by a professional with specific training to make this determination.

PSYCHOSIS. A mental disorder of emotional or organic origin characterized by personality derangement and loss of contact with reality.

QUADRIPLEGIC. Paralysis of all four extremities. This may be caused by spinal cord injury, but it can also be due to damage to both hemispheres of the brain.

RETENTION SPAN (MEMORY SPAN). The number of pieces of information heard or read that a person can retain at one time.

SPEECH PATHOLOGIST. Someone who has obtained an advanced degree in the profession of Speech Pathology, which deals with the study and treatment of all aspects of functional and organic speech and language disorders.

SPEECH OR LANGUAGE THERAPIST. Someone who has obtained the required training in the profession of Speech Pathology for treating disordered speech and/or language. In some situations these terms along with "speech pathologist" are used interchangeably, but strictly speaking there are differences.

THROMBO-EMBOLIC. Obstruction of a blood vessel due to thrombosis embolism, or both, as opposed to rupture of a blood vessel.

THROMBOSIS. A clot formed in a blood vessel that causes a narrowing and perhaps eventual total obstruction of that blood vessel.

TIA (pronounced as separate letters). *Transient Ischemic Attack*. An episode of neurological impairment which occurs abruptly and may last for minutes or hours—up to 24 hours—with eventual return to the preattack condition. Considered to be causally related to thromboembolism or sudden change in circulatory dynamics such as may occur with altered cardiac rhythm.

VASCULAR. This refers to the blood vessels which include the arteries, veins, and capillaries.

Bibliography

Broida, Helen. "Language Therapy Effects in Long Term Aphasia." *Archives of Physical Medicine and Rehabilitation* 58 (June 1977): 248-253.

Farrell, Barry. *Pat and Roald*. New York: Random House, 1969.

Fields, William S. "Cerebral Vascular Disease: Rehabilitation." in Fields, William S. (ed.) *Neurological and Sensory Disorders in the Elderly*. New York: Stratton Intercontinental Medical Book Corp., 1975. Selected papers and discussions from the Houston Neurological Symposium sponsored by the University of Texas Health Science Center at Houston.

Heslinga, K., Schellen, A. M. C. M., and Verkuyl, A. *Not Made of Stone: The Sexual Problems of Handicapped People*. Springfield: Charles C. Thomas, 1974.

Porch, Bruce E. *Porch Index of Communicative Ability*. Vol. II. Palo Alto: Consulting Psychologists Press, 1967.

Stryker, Stephanie. *Speech After Stroke: A Manual for the Speech Pathologist and the Family Member*. Springfield: Charles C. Thomas, 1975.

Wulf, Helen H. *Aphasia, My World Alone*. Detroit: Wayne State University Press, 1973. A personal account of recovery from aphasia.

Index

Activities of Daily Living (ADL); definition, 127; occupational therapy for, 70

American Heart Association, 123; for help with stroke clubs, 32; for locating day care centers or closed workshops, 105; for manuals, 101, 102, 125

American Speech and Hearing Association (ASHA), 123; for referrals, 24

Amyotropic Lateral Sclerosis (ALS) and dysarthria, 98

Aphasia, 1, 17, 18, 127; abstract ability in, 75; apraxia of speech and, 87; arithmetic and, 7, 18, 78-83 (See also Arithmetic impairment); automatic speech in, 47; bilingualism in, 40-41; card playing and, 83; catastrophic reactions in, 84; causes of, 5, 9, 18; communication notebook for, 58-59; concrete thinking and, 75; dementia and, 13-14, 128 (See also Dementia); driving ability and, 29-30, 108 (See also Driving ability with brain injury); dysarthria and, 7, 86-87 (See also Dysarthria); employment potential with, 6, 20, 105, 109; expressive, 37; fluent, 46-47; gestures, use of in, 7, 17, 33-34, 74-77 (See also Gestures, Pantomime and Signs); handedness and, 8, 15, 27, 70-71 (See also Handedness in Aphasia); hearing loss and, 37; home treatment of, 26-29, 41-43, 49-59, 64-67, 73, 76-79, 83-85; improvement potential of, 18-21; inconsistency of, 21-23; language skills disrupted in, 7; motor apraxia and, 75; naming objects in, 49, 53; number concepts and, 78-79; paralysis and (See Paralysis); patterns of speech problems in, 46-48; patterns of understanding speech in, 35-36, 38-40; perseveration in, 22, 47-48, 55, 128; plateauing of progress in, 20; processing time in, 38; profanity, use of in, 47-49; reading impairment in, 7, 18, 60-67; receptive, 37; sensory apraxia and, 75; sign language and, 75-76; singing, use of for 55; speech comprehension impairment in, 7, 18, 33-44; speech impairment in, 7, 17, 46-59; spontaneous improvement of, 19-20; symbolic ability in, 75; Stroke Clubs for, 30-32; telegraphic speech in, 46; telling patient of, 23; testing of (See Testing Aphasia); time concepts and, 83-84; treatment of (See Speech therapy for Aphasia); treatment, need for in, 19, 20, 23-26; understanding of patient's speech in, 53-55; word-finding problems in, 46; workbooks for treatment of, 28, 131; writing impairment in, 7, 18, 68-73; yes-no confusion in, 48

Apraxia; constructional, 70, 127; dementia and, 13, 75; motor, 75, 127; oral, 88, 89, 127; sensory, 13, 75, 127; of speech (See Apraxia of Speech)

Apraxia of Speech, 7, 86, 127; aphasia and, 87; causes of, 7; communication notebook for, 93; drawing and, 93; dysarthria and, 86-88, 91; expressive aphasia and, 87; gestures, use of with, 76, 93; home treatment for, 90-94; ice used for, 90; improvement potential for, 89-92; oral apraxia compared to, 88, 89; testing of, 87; treatment, need for early in, 20, 24-25, 89-91; typewriter used for, 27, 71; varieties of ability in, 88; writing and, 71, 93

Arithmetic impairment in aphasia, 7, 18, 78-85; calculation ability, 79-83; card playing and, 83; counting and, 78, 79; handling of finances and, 80-82; testing of impairment in, 78-85